MULTIPLE SCLEROSIS
A Guide for Patients and Their Families

Second Edition

MULTIPLE SCLEROSIS
A Guide for Patients and Their Families

Second Edition

Editor
Labe C. Scheinberg, M.D.
Professor of Neurology and Rehabilitation Medicine
Albert Einstein College of Medicine
Yeshiva University
Bronx, New York

Associate Editor
Nancy J. Holland, M.A., R.N.
Clinical Associate
Department of Neurology
Albert Einstein College of Medicine
Yeshiva University
Bronx, New York

Raven Press New York

Raven Press, 1185 Avenue of the Americas, New York, New York 10036

© 1987 by Raven Press Books, Ltd. All rights reserved. This book is protected by copyright. No part of it may be reproduced, stored in a retrieval system, or transmitted, in any form or by any means, electronic, mechanical, photocopying, recording, or otherwise, without the prior written permission of the publisher.

Made in the United States of America

Library of Congress Cataloging-in-Publication Data

Multiple sclerosis.

   Includes bibliographies and index.
   1. Multiple sclerosis. I. Scheinberg, Labe C.,
1925–   . II. Holland, Nancy J. [DNLM:
1. Multiple Sclerosis—popular works. W1 360 M9563]
RC377.M843   1987   616.8'34   86-29774
ISBN 0-88167-254-8
ISBN 0-88167-255-6 (soft)

   The material contained in this volume was submitted as previously unpublished material, except in the instances in which credit has been given to the source from which some of the illustrative material was derived.
   Great care has been taken to maintain the accuracy of the information contained in the volume. However, Raven Press cannot be held responsible for errors or for any consequences arising from the use of the information contained herein.

9 8 7 6 5 4 3 2 1

Dedication

Arthur Simon Abramson dedicated his life to improving on many levels the lives of the disabled. He was an educator, leader, investigator, and physician who was internationally recognized and active in many organizations. He brought a special depth of understanding to his work because of his own disability. This book is dedicated to him.

Dr. Abramson was born on June 4, 1912 in Montreal, Canada. He graduated from McGill University with a B.S. degree in 1934, and from McGill University Medical School in 1937.

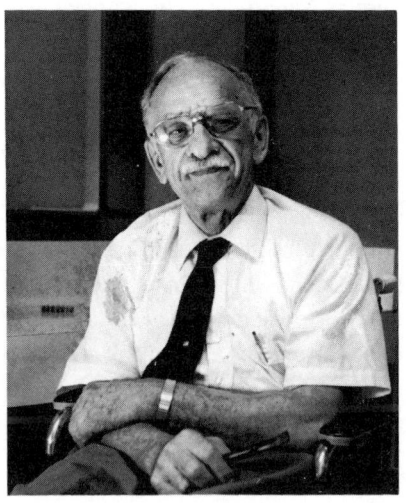

Arthur Simon Abramson
1912–1982

He came to the United States in 1938 as an intern at Newark Beth Israel Hospital, Newark, New Jersey. He returned to Montreal for his residency, but came to New York City in 1940 to specialize in orthopedic medicine at the Montefiore Hospital and then at the Hospital for Joint Diseases from 1941 to 1942.

On September 12, 1942, Dr. Abramson volunteered and was commissioned in the United States Army. He served in the European Theater in the 99th General Hospital as an orthopedic surgeon. During the Battle of the Bulge, on December 27, 1944, near Lyon, France, he was hit by a sniper's bullet, which caused paraplegia.

After many months of rehabilitation, he spent two years as a resident in Physical Medicine and Rehabilitation, becoming a diplomate in 1948. He continued as a physiatrist at the Bronx Veterans Hospital, becoming Chief of the Rehabilitation Service in 1950. During that time, he was clinical professor of Physical Medicine and Rehabilitation at New York Medical College. In 1955 he became the first Chairman of the Physical Medicine and Rehabilitation Department at the Albert Einstein College of Medicine, The Bronx, New York.

Dr. Abramson married in 1956, the same year he received the President's Award as Handicapped Man of the Year. He had a son in 1958.

In the early 1970s, he was the guiding force in the organization of the MS Comprehensive Care Center of the Albert Einstein College of Medicine, and taught by example as well as by word. His life was a model of courage and compassion for the disabled.

A "Disabled Bill of Rights," which he wrote, was his creed. He conducted significant research and treated patients throughout his entire professional life. Dr. Abramson achieved much for others, traveled the world, and worked until he died at the age of 70. He is missed, and we try to continue toward his dream.

Preface

Multiple sclerosis is the most common cause of neurological disability that attacks men and women between the ages of 15 and 55. Approximately 90% have their onset in this age range. It is rare to contract the condition before age 15 or after age 55. After trauma and arthritic disorders, multiple sclerosis is the most important cause of moderate to severe disability of adult life. Because of the long life expectancy associated with the disease, there are few, if any, conditions that have a greater socioeconomic impact. Often individuals are affected during the late stages of education and training or just as they have embarked on establishing a family and/or career. Generally multiple sclerosis strikes persons who are healthy, intelligent, and well educated—those to whom the future seems exceptionally bright. It cannot be attributed to any known "failing" or cause.

Multiple sclerosis is a chronic illness that can affect most motor and sensory functions of the nervous system. Pain and loss of mental faculties are rare. The disease varies in severity and allows some to lead full, productive lives, whereas others become severely disabled.

Although the cause of multiple sclerosis is unknown, it is thought to be the result of an abnormal response of the body to persistent infections. Much of the current research is directed along these lines. Moreover, there is no specific treatment, and nothing alters its unpredictable course. Attacks and remissions come without warning, confusing both patients and their families and making them prey to the many fad treatments that are always available in such circumstances.

Only through research into the cause and mechanism of symptom development can we hope to find a prevention or cure for this disease. This difficult and costly approach often seems inefficient, but as long as individuals are disabled, the search for a cure must continue. Sometimes answers come unexpectedly from seemingly unrelated fields within basic biomedical research; more often this route is slow and arduous.

In the meantime, health care teams continue to offer symptomatic treatment to the person with multiple sclerosis to prevent or alleviate painful, disabling, and potentially life-shortening complications. These teams also provide counseling and support to the affected person and his or her family. Moreover, there are enough resources in our society to carry on a forceful research program and to provide medically appropriate symptomatic treatment, particularly if these are not wasted on unproved therapies and quackery.

This book is intended as a guide for patients at any stage of the illness and for their families. It is a comprehensive, multidisciplinary approach, and those who have contributed to it have had long experience in dealing with the problems described herein.

Multiple sclerosis with its varied complications is frustrating to the patient, the family, and the health practitioner. However, through the consistent and cooperative effort of all three, in collaboration with the National Multiple Sclerosis Society and other interested agencies, the answers will come. Until that time, we must be increasingly concerned with better management of the day-to-day problems encountered by the person who has multiple sclerosis.

Sylvia Lawry
Founder–Director
National Multiple Sclerosis Society

Acknowledgments

The contributors wish to acknowledge the editorial assistance of Jeanne Fogg and Dr. Diana M. Schneider, and the secretarial assistance of Nancy Denner and Donna Maffia.

Royalties from the sale of this book are being contributed to support the educational, research, and patient care programs of the New York City Chapter of the National Multiple Sclerosis Society.

Contents

1 Introduction 1
   Labe C. Scheinberg

2 Epidemiology and Genetics of Multiple Sclerosis ... 3
   Charles M. Poser

3 What Causes the Disease? 13
   John N. Whitaker

4 The Diagnosis 25
   Charles M. Poser and Mindy Aisen

5 Signs and Symptoms of Multiple Sclerosis 43
   Labe C. Scheinberg and Charles R. Smith

6 Drug Therapy 53
   Labe C. Scheinberg and Barbara S. Giesser

7 Treatment with Diet 67
   James Q. Simmons and Barbara S. Giesser

8 Physical and Surgical Therapy 79
   Justin Alexander and Ellen Costello

9 Making Everyday Activities Easier 109
   Kate Robbins and Brian Rosenthal

10 Nursing Care 129
   Nancy J. Holland, Phyllis Wiesel-Levison, and Frances Francabandera

11 Bladder and Bowel Management 147
   Nancy J. Holland and Frances Francabandera

12 Sexuality 177
   Rosalind C. Kalb, Nicholas G. LaRocca, and Seymour R. Kaplan

13 Psychological Issues 197
   Nicholas G. LaRocca, Rosalind C. Kalb, and Seymour R. Kaplan

| 14 | Social Adaptations | 215 |

Nancy J. Holland and Seymour R. Kaplan

| 15 | Vocational Issues | 229 |

Nancy J. Holland, Seymour R. Kaplan, and
Harry L. Hall

| 16 | What About New Treatments? | 239 |

Robert J. Slater and Labe C. Scheinberg

| 17 | Available Services | 247 |

Diann Geronemus

Subject Index 261

Contributors

Mindy Aisen, M.D.
Department of Neurology
Albert Einstein College of Medicine
1300 Morris Park Avenue
Bronx, NY 10461

Justin Alexander, Ph.D.
Department of Rehabilitation
  Medicine
Albert Einstein College of Medicine
1300 Morris Park Avenue
Bronx, NY 10461

Ellen Costello, P.T., M.S.
Division of Physical Therapy
Ithaca College, Bronx Campus
Albert Einstein College of Medicine
1300 Morris Park Avenue
Bronx, NY 10461

Frances Francabandera, MSN, R.N.
Medical Rehabilitation Research and
  Training for MS
Albert Einstein College of Medicine
1300 Morris Park Avenue
Bronx, NY 10461

Diann Geronemus, MSW, ACSW
Consultant
National Multiple Sclerosis Society
2700 Southwest 4th Avenue
Fort Lauderdale, FL 33315

Barbara S. Giesser, M.D.
Department of Neurology
Albert Einstein College of Medicine
1300 Morris Park Avenue
Bronx, NY 10461

Harry L. Hall
The Development Team, Inc.
4214 9th Street, North
Arlington, VA 22203

Nancy J. Holland, M.A., R.N.
Department of Neurology
Albert Einstein College of Medicine
1300 Morris Park Avenue
Bronx, NY 10461

Chris Holzer
Illustrator
141 Morris Turnpike
Randolph, NJ 07869

Rosalind Kalb, Ph.D.
Departments of Neurology and
  Rehabilitation Medicine
Albert Einstein College of Medicine
1300 Morris Park Avenue
Bronx, NY 10461

Seymour R. Kaplan, M.D.
Department of Psychiatry
Albert Einstein College of Medicine
1300 Morris Park Avenue
Bronx, NY 10461

CONTRIBUTORS

Nicholas G. LaRocca, Ph.D.
Department of Neurology
(Psychology)
Albert Einstein College of Medicine
1300 Morris Park Avenue
Bronx, NY 10461

Sylvia Lawry
National Multiple Sclerosis Society
205 East 42nd Street
New York, NY 10017

Charles M. Poser, M.D.
Department of Neurology
Harvard Medical School
Beth Israel Hospital
Boston, MA 02215

Kate Robbins, M.A., OTR
Medical Rehabilitation Research and
 Training Center for MS
Albert Einstein College of Medicine
1300 Morris Park Avenue
Bronx, NY 10461

Brian Rosenthal, M.D.
Department of Rehabilitation
 Medicine
Albert Einstein College of Medicine
1300 Morris Park Avenue
Bronx, NY 10461

Labe Scheinberg, M.D.
Department of Neurology and
 Rehabilitation Medicine
Albert Einstein College of Medicine
1300 Morris Park Avenue
Bronx, NY 10461

James Simmons, M.D.
(Deceased)
Consultant
National Multiple Sclerosis Society
205 East 42nd Street
New York, NY 10017

Robert J. Slater, M.D.
National Multiple Sclerosis Society
205 East 42nd Street
New York, NY 10017

Charles Smith, M.D.
Department of Neurology
Albert Einstein College of Medicine
1300 Morris Park Avenue
Bronx, NY 10461

John Whitaker, M.D.
Department of Neurology
University of Alabama at Birmingham
OHB-358 University Station
Birmingham, AL 35294

Phyllis Wiesel-Levison, B.S., R.N.
Medical Rehabilitation Research and
 Training Center for MS
Albert Einstein College of Medicine
1300 Morris Park Avenue
Bronx, NY 10461

MULTIPLE SCLEROSIS
A Guide for Patients and Their Families

Second Edition

1

Introduction

Labe C. Scheinberg

Multiple sclerosis is a chronic, sometimes disabling disease of the central nervous system; it is almost always confusing and frustrating to the patients and their families. The diagnosis may be learned only after repeated examinations, and the response may be a sense of dread or in many cases one of relief after long periods of uncertainty and concern that the cause of the symptoms might have been even worse or psychogenic. Frequently it is a new term to the patient and family. When they are familiar with it, they know it only from the worst cases so obvious because of the severe disability. If not familiar, they seek information from books, which often give a preponderantly pessimistic prognosis. The physician in this busy world may not be available for detailed explanation at the moment or to answer questions, so many of which arise after the initial shock has worn off.

This book is written for the patient and family, something to be read on learning the diagnosis or to be read at various times in the course of the illness to help understand what is happening and explain how to deal with it. Multiple sclerosis is a variable disease in its severity, and this book is written for the mildest case, who may enjoy a full active life of normal expectancy, as well as for the severe case, who rapidly becomes disabled.

The organization of this book is traditional, beginning with a section on the possible causes (etiologies) and development (pathogenesis) of multiple sclerosis (MS). Current hypotheses concerning the origin of MS are presented along with possible contributing factors. The remaining sections are more clinical, with a discussion of diagnosis and management by medical, surgical, physical, and psychological methods. The patients' problems are foremost, whether these are questions of diet, employment, sex, physical therapy, social adaptation, or unproved therapies.

If one were asked for a brief description of MS, one could probably best reply, "It is an unpredictable neurological disorder (disease of the nervous system) with its onset in early adult life, mostly affecting walking, and often with associated urinary problems." There are, of course, visual and other sensory symptoms, fatigue, psychological problems, sexual difficulties, etc., but the major disability is in the area of mobility. When patients are asked what is their major problem, 90% will respond "Difficulty in walking." All of these problems are discussed in detail.

Multiple sclerosis is common enough to have earned the title of "the great crippler of young adults." Although the exact number of cases in the United States is unknown, it must approximate 200,000. After arthritis and trauma, it is the chief cause of major disability in adults of working age, that is, those between 16 and 60. The overall economic, social, and psychosexual implications are overwhelming in many instances. Because MS strikes individuals in their most productive years, just when they are assuming major family and career responsibilities, its impact may be greater than that of any other physical illness.

2

Epidemiology and Genetics of Multiple Sclerosis

Charles M. Poser

EPIDEMIOLOGY

Epidemiology is the study of the distribution of disease in human populations in different countries and localities and of the factors that affect their characteristics. It is concerned with circumstances that might contribute to causing or aggravating a disease, its sex and family distribution, the areas of the world or countries that have a high incidence of the disease, and which ethnic groups are more frequently affected by it.

Although epidemiologic studies have traditionally been thought helpful mainly in the study of infectious diseases, a little over 30 years ago these methods began to be applied to multiple sclerosis (MS). Many studies have been carried out.

The results of these studies should be considered with great caution for the following reasons: the diagnosis of MS is strictly a clinical one, and therefore it is dependent on the skill of the researchers who carried out the study; not all of these investigators, who work independently, use the same diagnostic criteria, so that results in one group may not be exactly comparable with a group taken elsewhere; it is not possible to be sure of having identified all cases of the disease in a particular geographic area. Not to be forgotten are many other factors that may influence the results of the study, such as the availability and the sophistication of medical personnel and the fact that MS patients might relocate in an area where climatic conditions are more favorable and medical care more easily available.

Two terms need to be defined since they are commonly used in epidemiologic reports. The first one is *incidence,* which means the number of new cases of a disease that are diagnosed during a particular period of time, usually a calendar year, in a defined geographic area such as a country, a county, or a city, and reported in terms of a unit of population, usually per 100,000 people. Thus, if a report states that the incidence of MS in a country is 7/100,000, this means that during the specified year seven cases were newly discovered per 100,000 population; if it is a country of 4 million people, this would mean that during that one year there were 280 new cases of the disease. On the other hand, the term *prevalence* refers to the number of patients with MS who are identified on a particular day in a defined geographic area, also expressed in terms of a unit of population. Thus, in the same country, a count of the actual number of MS patients living there on the 19th of April, 1984, may result in a prevalence of 30/100,000, which is another way of saying that 1,200 patients were identified.

It is evident from this that when epidemiologic surveys deal with small populations, the addition or subtraction of a single case may mean a great difference. This has been a major problem in attempting to evaluate both incidence and prevalence studies.

These difficulties notwithstanding, it is generally accepted that MS is more common in countries farther from the equator, both in the northern and southern hemispheres (Fig. 1). It is encountered considerably more frequently in Great Britain, the Scandinavian countries, and northern Germany than in the countries around the Mediterranean sea. It is more common in Canada and the northern tier of the United States than in the southern areas of the country (see Table 1).

Unfortunately, very little information is available from vast areas such as Latin America, most of Asia, and the Soviet Union. Other well-established epidemiologic data have shown that the disease is quite rare among Orientals (in particular the Japanese), and it has never been diagnosed convincingly among black Africans. In American blacks, the disease is somewhat less common than in nonblacks but

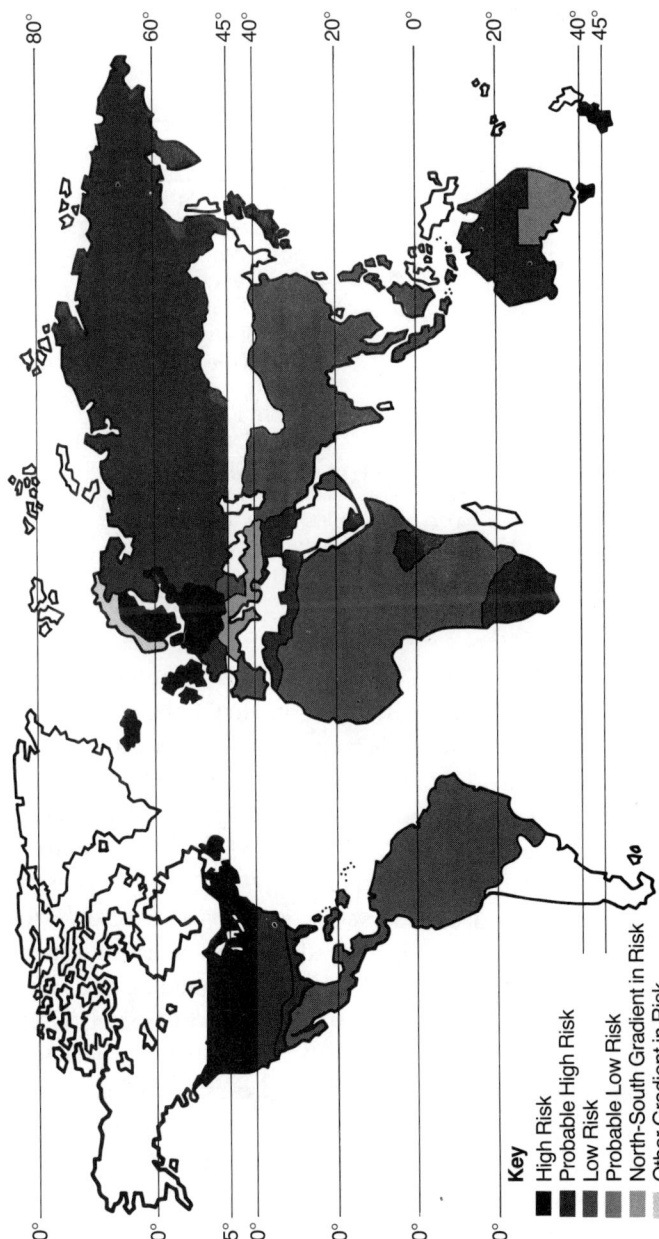

FIG. 1. World map indicating MS incidence. (Modified by National Institute of Neurological and Communicative Disorders and Stroke: Multiple sclerosis: hope through research, No. 79-75, Washington, D.C., 1981, National Institutes of Health.)

TABLE 1. *Prevalence and latitude*

Latitude	Prevalence (per 100,000)	City/country
65° N	72	Iceland
61° N	129	Shetland Islands
59° N	108	Orkney Islands
44° N	64	Rochester, MN
44° N	11	Yugoslavia
44° N	9	Arles, France
43° S	32	Hobart, Tasmania
43° N	2	Sapporo, Japan
42° N	41	Boston, MA
42° N	6	Bulgaria
38° N	30	San Francisco, CA
38° N	2	Seoul, Korea
33° N	14	Charleston, SC
33° S	20	Newcastle, Australia
32° N	0.7	Iran and Iraq
30° N	6	New Orleans, LA
30° S	38	South Australia

shows the same gradient related to latitude: it is more common in blacks living in Boston than in those living in New Orleans.

Recent studies seem to show higher rates of MS than earlier ones, probably as a result of more thorough evaluation, longer survival because of better treatment, and more accurate diagnosis. There is no evidence to suggest that there has been an actual increase in the frequency of the disease despite these reports.

In reviewing the incidence and prevalence of the disease in the northern latitudes, it should be remembered that these areas have been settled overwhelmingly by persons of Germanic (including Scandinavian and Anglo-Saxon) origin, those often referred to as the "North Sea people." This is also true of South Africa, Australia, and New Zealand. It appears that in these populations (i.e., those of Germanic ancestry), location, i.e., the more northern and more southern latitudes, determines the risk. This explains why the rates of MS in North America (with its predominantly North Sea population) are substantially higher than those in Europe at similar latitudes (with predominantly individuals of Mediterranean origin). Interestingly, differences in latitude do not seem to influence the incidence or prevalence of the disease among Orientals and American Indians and Eskimos. In Asia and Africa, similarly, the incidence appears to be low regardless of latitude.

All of these well-documented studies lead to the conclusion that Caucasians of northern and central European origin appear to be genetically susceptible, but their geographic location, i.e., the environment, affects the risk of actually developing the disease. It is the necessary combination of genetic susceptibility and an environmental factor, possibly geographic in nature, as well as other factors that result in the eventual acquisition of MS.

The biological significance of latitude has remained mysterious. There is no evidence that it is related to climate. Studies with mixed and inconsistent results have suggested that the disease is more common in countries that have achieved high levels of industrialization, sanitation, and a high standard of living. Studies in England have reported a predilection of the disease for the socially fortunate, but similar studies in other countries have not confirmed this. On the other hand, the disease is not related to poverty, overcrowding, or other indices of low socioeconomic status. The risk of urban versus rural environment is unclear.

Studies of persons who have migrated from one area to another have shown that migration from a high-risk area (northern Europe) to a low-risk area (Israel or South Africa) before puberty is associated with a reduction in the risk of MS. On the other hand, among the descendants of these immigrants to Israel, the environment appears to extend a protective effect to those descendants of Jewish immigrants from northern and eastern Europe and a possible reverse effect for the descendants of those who came from Africa and Asia. Insufficient data are available to determine the effect of the reverse type of migration, from low-risk (the West Indies or Indochina) to high-risk areas (London or Paris). Usually, however, such migrants are non-Caucasians, who do not appear to have the same genetic susceptibility to the disease.

Certain areas of the world have been identified as having unexpectedly high incidence and prevalence. These include the Shetland and Orkney Islands to the northeast of Scotland, certain areas in Norway, small areas in Sicily, and even Key West, Florida, and small towns such as Duxbury and Mansfield, Massachusetts. The significance, if any, of these findings is unknown, but these reports have all been about very small populations, where the addition of a single case has an enormous statistical impact of dubious biological significance.

It has even been suggested that epidemics of MS have occurred, leading some investigators to propose that the disease is a transmissible one, meaning that it may be contagious. Such an "epidemic" has been reported in the Faroe Islands and believed to have been the result of, or at least related to, the fact that the islands were occupied by British troops during the years 1940–1945. Similarly, an "epidemic" was believed to have occurred in Iceland after Canadian and U.S. troops were stationed there. These findings, however, were based on the clinical appearance of the disease, which does not correspond to the actual onset of the illness, which most probably had been acquired several years before. In fact, based on the immigration studies to Israel and South Africa, several researchers have concluded that the disease begins between the ages of 5 and 15, or before puberty. When the data from which the "epidemics" in the Faroes and in Iceland are recalculated on this basis, it becomes apparent that there was no epidemic at all.

Despite the immigration data, there is absolutely no evidence to support the idea that migration from a high-risk to a low-risk area would in any way affect the development of the disease in a person who already has acquired it. The idea that individuals in whose close family MS has been diagnosed might avoid developing the disease by migrating to a low-risk area before puberty has never been tested, but studies in twins, where concordance (both twins having MS) is low, makes such a possibility improbable.

The sum of epidemiologic information in general supports the idea that the disease is the result of the combination of genetic factors expressed most likely as an inherited susceptibility that is affected by environmental factors that to this date remain unidentified; viral infections are strongly suspected to play an important role in initiating the disease process.

Because many MS patients have high level of antibodies against measles and other viruses in their blood, the view that infections such as measles play an important role in causing a susceptible individual to develop MS has gained support. It should be pointed out, however, that the siblings of MS patients who do not have the disease have similarly high titers of antibodies against measles and several other viruses. Nevertheless, for the past several years attempts have been made to relate the development of MS to exposure to dogs, in particular pointing to the fact that a common disease of these animals, canine distemper, is caused by a virus of the measles family. The results of many studies have been quite contradictory and inconsistent.

For many years investigators have searched for a single virus causing MS. The search has been fruitless, and it is quite probable that it will remain so. Multiple sclerosis is not an infection. The extreme rarity of conjugal cases (man and wife both having MS) and the small number of cases occurring in the same household do not indicate a contagious factor.

Despite these inconsistencies, it is likely that a nonspecific, probably viral, infection brings out the disease in a genetically susceptible person. Thus, in one individual MS might develop secondary to measles, in another one to chickenpox, and in a third one to one of the many varieties of influenza.

GENETIC FACTORS

One of the major results of the epidemiologic studies has been the repeated confirmation that genetic factors play an important role in the development of MS. It has already been mentioned that the disease is unusual in Orientals, unknown in African blacks, and less frequent in American blacks. It is considerably less common in individuals of Hispanic origin than in those of Germanic, Anglo-Saxon, and Scandinavian origin. Multiple sclerosis is also more common in women than men (1.5 : 1), suggesting a possible but unknown hormonal influence. The disease does occur in families, and siblings have six to eight times the risk of acquiring the disease. These figures, however, apply only to families in high-susceptibility ethnic groups. Surprisingly, however, studies of twins show that there is a very low rate of concordance (both members of the twin pair having the disease), which has been interpreted as favoring an environmental factor rather than a genetic one. The exact nature of the genetic factor remains unknown.

In the "North Sea" populations, certain characteristics of the histocompatibility system (HLA) are more frequently observed and statistically significant in MS patients than in non-MS controls. The histocompatibility system is that part of the immune system that controls the acceptance or rejection of tissue transplants such as skin grafts, kidneys, or other organs. Several studies show that in Caucasian MS patients in the United States, Canada, Scandinavia, and Australia there is a significant statistical difference between MS patients and controls for the histocompatibility factors A3, B7, DW2, and DR2. On the other hand, these factors are not found in Israeli or Japanese MS patients despite the fact that the disease in those individuals is no different than in other people. Furthermore, in studies of families in which two or three members have the disease, the results are inconsistent: the MS patients may share these HLA factors, but just as frequently they do not, whereas non-MS members of the family similarly may have these same factors without having developed the disease. Determining these histocompatibility factors will not provide any prognostic information to siblings or other close blood relatives of MS patients. Unfortunately, this practice is carried out in some medical centers despite the fact that the results are clinically worthless. The genetic susceptibility to the disease is almost certainly not related to the histocompatibility system; the genetic traits are probably transmitted by a different mechanism.

CONCLUSION

The only conclusions that can now be drawn from both epidemiologic and genetic studies are as follows: there appears to be a genetic susceptibility to the disease that is highest in descendants of "North Sea people"; this genetic susceptibility is not related to the histocompatibility system; MS patients and their siblings seem to share the genetic trait of having immune systems that respond very actively to various infections by producing high titers of antibodies; an environmental factor, probably an infection, affecting the individual between the ages of 5 and 15 (or puberty) seems necessary for "activating" the genetic susceptibility.

Until now neither epidemiologic nor genetic studies have reached the level of practical, clinical significance, although they will continue to provide important clues to the developmental mechanisms of the disease.

3

What Causes the Disease?

John N. Whitaker

Multiple sclerosis (MS) is a disease in which the insulation surrounding nerve fibers of the central nervous system (the brain and spinal cord) is damaged. Tissue outside the central nervous system is not involved in the disease. Infections of the urinary and respiratory systems, which are commonly seen in persons with MS, are simply complications of MS.

Although knowledge about the factors influencing the development of MS has increased appreciably during the last decade, its cause is basically unknown. We can speculate, however, and offer here some possible causes. In addition, the basic damage that occurs within the body must be understood so that the MS individual and his or her family can better cope with the disorder.

WHY THE SYMPTOMS?

In order to identify the pathological changes that explain the symptoms in patients with MS, it is necessary to understand some of the anatomy of the central nervous system (CNS). This system is characterized by the specialized activities of its component cells. Actions and reactions of the individual's body depend on "news" of the stimulus being transmitted to the brain, the brain's reaction, and "instructions" on how to react to the stimulus then being sent from the brain back to the original point. This coordinated transmission of a nerve impulse from one nerve cell to the next underlies nervous tissue function and is dependent on the connections among the nerve cells. These "connections'' are called nerve fibers. The coordination among these nerve cells is a result of the integrity (intactness) and the speed of conduction of an impulse along the nerve fiber to the synapse (connection point) to the next nerve cell. Myelin (a fatty substance that surrounds the nerve fiber, forming a sheath) is made and maintained by a cell called the oligodendrocyte and enhances the velocity with which nerve impulses are conducted along the fibers.

The conduction of an impulse along an axon (the nerve fiber leading to the synapse) may be viewed as similar to the movement of current in an electrical wire (Fig. 1). Myelin provides the insulation around nerve fibers and allows only a small portion of the nerve fiber membrane (at the node of Ranvier) to become depolarized (change in electrical charge) and the impulse to be transmitted. The presence of the myelin sheath markedly reduces any leakage of "current."

In MS this sheath is damaged, so that the insulation can no longer prevent leakage (Fig. 2). As a result, transmission may either be delayed or cease completely. In either event, a nervous system activity (such as vision, strength, sensation, or coordination) is diminished or lost because of the delay or block in impulse transmission.

The initial lesion (area of abnormality) in MS that leads to the tissue alterations (myelin damage) is still unclear (Fig. 3). However, it is known that oligodendrocytes are altered or damaged and myelin breaks down in the presence of cells from the immune system invading the CNS. As the myelin is damaged, certain other cells proliferate and form dense tissue at the site of the damage. This proliferation causes a firmness of the tissue (sclerosis). Sclerotic tissue is similar to scar tissue. The loss of myelin, the sclerosis, and the fact that the lesions (often referred to as plaques) occur in many sites throughout the CNS account for the name "multiple" or "disseminated" sclerosis. The water content of the plaques increases, which permits their detection by magnetic resonance imaging.

There are areas of inflammation in MS that are usually characterized by the accumulation of cells, especially in the early phases of the disease; these cells usually accumulate around blood vessels in the CNS (Fig. 4). It is not known how or why they arrive at the site where they eventually gather and form a lesion. It is known, however,

CAUSES

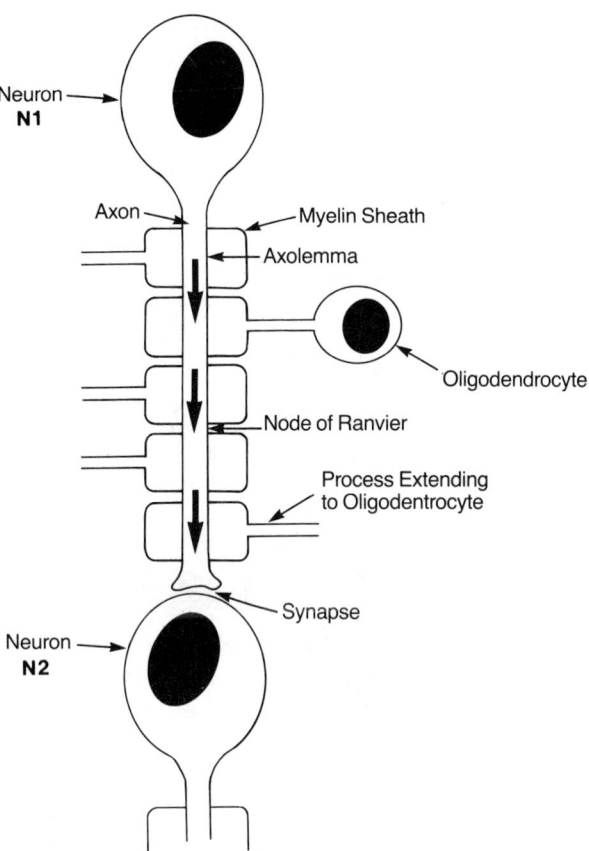

FIG. 1. Two neurons (N1 and N2) are depicted separated by a synapse in normal CNS tissue. The nerve impulse (thick arrow) travels down the axon and is prevented from leaking outward through the axolemma (the extension from the neuron) by the insulation provided by the myelin sheath, which in turn is made by and nourished by the oligodendrocyte. Only at the node of Ranvier is the area of the axolemma normally not covered by the myelin sheath.

CAUSES

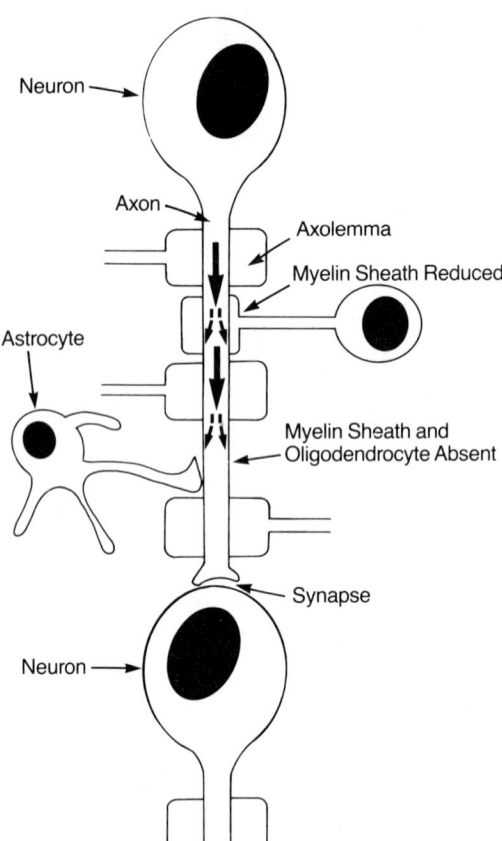

FIG. 2. In MS, the neuron, axon, axolemma, and synapse remain intact, but the myelin sheath is damaged or lost, and the oligodendrocytes are reduced in number. The reduction in the thickness of the myelin sheath permits part of the nerve impulse (thick arrow) to leak outward (thin arrow with dashed lines) through the axolemma, leading to a delay in nerve impulse transmission. This might give rise, if it is located in the nerve for vision, to slight blurring of vision. When the myelin sheath is absent, nerve impulse transmission stops, leading to a conduction block. If a conduction block were present in the nerve for vision, this would result in blindness. Astrocytes increase in number and size, possibly attaching to the axolemma and preventing regeneration of the myelin sheath.

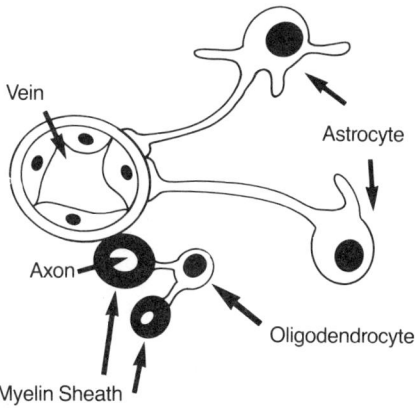

FIG. 3. This figure shows some of the same normal structures depicted in Fig. 1. The axon, surrounded by the myelin sheath, which in turn is supported by the oligodendrocyte, is shown along with the vein, which contains blood involved in providing nutrients for cells. Also shown is the normal astrocyte.

that they both injure the tissue and digest (phagocytize) the damaged myelin. The cells that phagocytize the myelin are macrophages.

Another cell that appears to be related to this inflammatory collection, but which remains within the CNS for a long period of time, is the plasma cell. This cell produces immunoglobulin, which is a protein in the serum that contains antibodies. The plasma cells found within brain tissue of persons with MS may produce large amounts of immunoglobulin (previously referred to as gammaglobulin). Because this material may then spill into the cerebrospinal fluid and its presence can be detected by laboratory tests, its presence is used to help in the diagnosis of MS.

The damage to myelin in nerve cells, which is seen when tissues are examined after death, is usually more extensive than was suggested by the symptoms seen during life. Hence, it appears that there are attacks in patients that have not produced symptoms severe enough to be felt by the patient or seen by the doctor. That these subclinical attacks occur means that there is yet no clear way to predict the course of tissue injury in this disease, as the extent of the damage can be seen only after death.

18   CAUSES

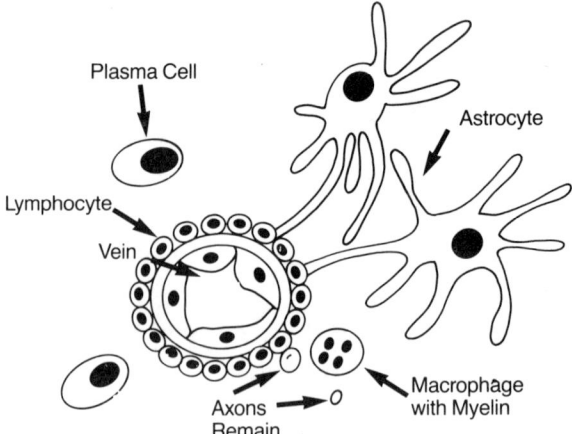

FIG. 4. In the area of damage in an MS plaque, lymphocytes surround blood vessels, usually veins, and lead to damage and loss of myelin. The damaged myelin is engulfed by macrophages, also coming from blood. The axons, with their thinned or absent myelin sheaths, remain, and oligodendrocytes are reduced in number or absent. Some of the lymphocytes that enter the brain become plasma cells and make large amounts of antibody, which may enter cerebrospinal fluid and can be detected by a spinal tap. It is these plasma cells that give rise to the increase in immunoglobulin and oligoclonal bands of immunoglobulin in cerebrospinal fluid. The astrocytes enlarge in size and develop more processes, leading to scarring or sclerosis. This sclerosis occurs in many parts of the central nervous system (brain and spinal cord) and gives rise to the term MS.

WHAT CAUSES THE DAMAGE?

The basic features of MS were described over 100 years ago. Those observations and the ones made subsequently that have bearing on the cause of MS may be summarized as follows: MS is an acquired, inflammatory, primary breakdown of certain tissues in the CNS that occurs in multiple and random sites. Cellular overgrowth and a fibrotic response within these areas account for the sclerosis. It is uncertain how the disease then progresses, although we know that there is often subclinical involvement that goes undetected by the patient or on clinical examination. No absolutely specific diagnostic tests are yet available. There are also adjunctive methods involving X-ray-like imaging (such as magnetic resonance) of the brain and spinal cord, evoked potentials to measure how rapidly the visual, sound, and skin sensations travel in the nervous system, and tests of cerebrospinal fluid to aid in the diagnosis. There are now procedures that measure certain components in the cerebrospinal fluid that indicate recent tissue damage and immunological studies that provide an indication about the mechanism.

As to the factors responsible for producing MS or, for that matter, any disorder for which the cause is unknown, the epidemiology (possible environmental influences) and genetics (possible susceptibility of the person who develops the disease) should be considered. The epidemiology and genetics of MS are considered in detail in Chapter 2. The results are consistent with some form of infectious agent acting on a person who is more predisposed or susceptible, with this susceptibility related to the immune system.

The epidemiology observed for MS suggests that viruses, toxins, or nutritional deficiency could be factors in the disease. Although a number of toxins (poisons) and certain vitamin-deficiency states may lead to nerve damage, the abnormal alterations in the CNS caused by these agents are different from those seen in MS; moreover, in these conditions there are often changes in the peripheral nervous system that do not occur in MS. There is no direct evidence that an environmental pollutant causes MS or that vitamins are in any way active in the prevention or arrest of MS. In terms of the environment, then, the strongest candidate is an infectious agent.

At what point in MS genetic factors are involved is unknown, but this is obviously an important question. The chromosome sites that determine which HLA types (the control of tissue type or uniqueness) are present lie near the genes that control the immune response (see the next section). Hence, a genetic influence could be related to an immune response to an infectious agent or to the body's autoimmune response to a substance within itself that the body (for some unknown reason) suddenly decides is not acceptable.

Thus, the etiology or cause of MS remains uncertain. The pathogenesis of MS, that is, the steps by which the myelin is damaged, involves the immune system. The remainder of this chapter considers the changes related to the immune system in MS.

THE IMMUNE SYSTEM

An "immune response" in any individual, with or without a specific disease, simply refers to the body reacting to a foreign agent (virus, bacteria, etc.) to protect itself against that agent. Occasionally the body goes "haywire" and starts to react against its own tissues. This is called an "autoimmune response."

The host's immune system may be involved in the onset or perpetuation of MS. Cells of lymphoid tissue (thymus, spleen, lymph nodes, certain blood cells) generate and control an immune response. In humans, most of the information has been obtained from studies of lymphocytes (certain blood cells), which are readily accessible for analysis. These lymphocytes may be subdivided into different types, which have several specialized functions. Some (B cells) produce and secrete antibody. Other lymphocytes (T cells) directly attack and destroy an infectious organism; these are "effector" T cells. Other T cells help promote an immune response or suppress it; these are "regulatory" T cells.

Investigation of the general immune status of persons with MS has disclosed no consistent abnormality in the blood, although when more specific and sensitive tests are used, regulatory lymphocytes of the T-suppressor type sometimes have been found to be reduced in number or action. That is, there may be a decrease or disappearance of these lymphocytes from the peripheral blood or a decline in their function at the very time MS exacerbates. The function of these cells returns to normal or above normal when the patient goes into remission. Whether these cells are destroyed, enter the CNS, or merely alter their circulatory route in the body remains to be determined. The lymphocytes in MS plaques (Fig. 3) include B and T lymphocytes without a selective T-cell type (helper or suppressor) dominant. It is also unclear how an alteration of the number of regulatory T lymphocytes would manifest as MS, but the correlation sometimes noted of the cyclic changes in clinical symptoms and the number of these cells in the bloodstream is intriguing.

Cerebrospinal Fluid

It has been known for more than 35 years that there is usually an increase in the amount of immunoglobulin in the cerebrospinal fluid of persons with MS. IgG is the predominant immunoglobulin.

Cerebrospinal fluid normally contains up to 45 milligrams of protein per 100 milliliters; IgG constitutes less than 15% of the total amount of protein present. As noted, in persons with MS, the IgG in the cerebrospinal fluid is increased, primarily because of the production of IgG by certain cells (plasma cells) (Fig. 4) within the CNS. These cells appear to arise from blood lymphocytes, which enter the CNS when the MS patient is having bouts of inflammatory myelin damage. When examined by suitable techniques, the cerebrospinal fluid proteins of the vast majority (80 to 90%) of persons with MS show selective increase of certain forms of IgG, but the presence of these forms of IgG in cerebrospinal fluid is not specific for MS; they are found in other diseases as well. In association with the changes in IgG in the cerebrospinal fluid, antibodies to a number of viruses are also found to be increased. However, neither of these conditions is specific for MS or even precisely parallels the disease's activity. The activity of the major part of the IgG in cerebrospinal fluid is unknown. Attempts to determine this activity are currently being made in many research laboratories.

VIRUSES AND MS

Viruses or other infectious agents have been suspected for many years to be the cause of MS. As different infectious organisms have been discovered and identified, they have been examined for a possible linkage to MS. During the past 20 years, attention to an infectious basis for MS has been directed primarily at viruses.

Numerous types of virus exist with an array of features that determine how they infect and alter tissue. The behavior of the virus is the result of a virus's own characteristics and the cells to which it is exposed. A host cell may show a number of reactions in response to a viral infection, ranging from minimal or no change to malignant transformation to death. In addition to the changes produced by the usual type of virus, mutant viruses may appear that have different characteristics of infectivity or disease induction.

Evidence for viral involvement in MS or any condition can be sought using several methods. The most convincing is the culture, isolation, and identification of a virus in tissues taken from areas of damage. Other methods include recognizing parts of a virus in tissue and detecting antibodies (which would attack that particular virus) in the blood or cerebrospinal fluid of those affected. Finding the antibody would indicate that the person had been exposed to the virus at one time or another.

The virus that causes measles (ruleola) has been analyzed extensively as a possible cause of MS. This measles virus is known also to cause a chronic nervous system disease of childhood called subacute sclerosing panencephalitis. Beginning in 1962, it was recognized that persons with MS have increased amounts of antibody to the measles virus in their bloodstream. Although a number of studies have confirmed this observation and have also shown that some of the antibody to measles is being produced by the CNS, evidence for the measles virus also causing MS remains highly circumstantial.

Dogs and MS

Even less convincing than the information on measles is the relationship between exposure to dogs and the development of MS. This is an emotional and highly controversial issue on which opinions differ. Canine distemper is a viral infection that produces an inflammatory disease of the CNS in dogs, and the canine distemper virus has a number of characteristics in common with the measles virus. Even though the case for incriminating dogs and/or canine distemper in the development of MS is unproven, an effective program for the vaccination of dogs against canine distemper should be followed.

Slow Virus

When attempting to relate environmental influences (see Chapter 2) from 10 to 20 years before to the appearance of MS now, a "slow virus" must be considered. In contrast to the usual acute or subacute response to conventional viruses, "slow viruses" cause diseases that may evolve over a period of months to years. One of these viruses induces an inflammatory CNS disease in sheep, but there is no indication that any one of the known "slow viruses" causes MS.

Other Viruses

Several conventional viruses have been identified as causing a CNS disease in animals that shows some of the same tissue changes as are seen in MS. Hence, because of the many mechanisms whereby a virus might inflict CNS damage, a viral etiology for MS has by no means been excluded.

Multiple Sclerosis: A Guide for Patients and Their Families, Second Edition, edited by L. C. Scheinberg and N. J. Holland. Raven Press © 1987.

4

The Diagnosis

Charles M. Poser and Mindy Aisen

Although some helpful diagnostic procedures and tests have been developed, the diagnosis of MS is still based on the history and neurological examination. The physician must be able to show that there are two or more areas of involvement (scars or lesions) of the central nervous system (the brain and spinal cord), that these lesions predominantly involve the white matter of the brain, and that other illnesses that also produce multiple abnormalities have been ruled out. There should be evidence that the lesions are disseminated not only in space (i.e., in different locations, e.g., optic nerve and spinal cord) but in time (symptoms or signs should develop at different times). Depending largely on the severity and duration of the disease, these findings can vary from being relatively easy to extremely difficult to confirm.

The diagnosis remains essentially a clinical one, based on symptoms and signs of the individual's nervous system malfunction. It is, therefore, highly dependent on the accuracy of the individual's medical history and on the physician's skill in eliciting and properly evaluating this information.

A *symptom* is something that is reported by the patient. Examples include diminished or abnormal sensation, weakness of a body part, a decrease in vision, or clumsiness. A *sign* is an abnormality detected by the physician while examining the person. At times, signs confirm the presence of symptoms. For example, a physician may be able to detect the weakness or delineate the sensory loss of which the patient complains. On the other hand, abnormal nervous system signs such as nystagmus (a jerking movement of the eyes,) abnormal reflexes such as the Babinski sign (when the sole of the foot is scratched, the big toe extends), or loss of vibratory sense may be present without the patient being aware of anything being wrong. Symptoms are subjective complaints, whereas signs are objective observations. The patient must search his or her memory and often turn to friends and close relatives in order to recall symptoms that may be significant. Finally, the physician may select certain procedures and laboratory tests that confirm that the patient does indeed have a medical abnormality that causes his or her symptoms. These various tests may provide evidence of the existence of multiple abnormal areas (lesions) in the nervous system.

PROBLEMS OF CLINICAL DIAGNOSIS

There are many difficulties inherent in the recall of symptoms by the individual and their interpretation by the doctor before a diagnosis of MS can be established. Symptoms may be decidedly transient, lasting not just hours or days but sometimes only minutes. They are often bizarre and so may be dismissed as irrelevant or not significant by both patient and physician. Because symptoms may be mild and fleeting, they are often easily forgotten.

Although information on the symptoms of MS is easily available to the public in specially prepared materials, many physicians, even neurologists, have little experience with this disease and so misinterpret the symptoms and sometimes make incorrect diagnoses. Medical terminology is often confusing both for the person affected and the physician. Other diseases that are called by the term "sclerosis" are sometimes confused with MS; for example, many people think that MS is the same as amyotrophic lateral sclerosis (Lou Gehrig's disease or motor neuron disease), although the two diseases have nothing in common whatsoever. The most common symptoms of MS are well known: numbness and tingling of an arm(s) or leg(s), double or blurred vision, fatigue, clumsiness of fine movements or of walking, and frequency and urgency of urination.

Unfortunately, many of these symptoms arise for other reasons. Blurring or graying of vision occurs far more often as a result of eye disease than it does because of the optic nerve inflammation (optic nerve neuritis) that is characteristic of MS. True double vision (which is common in MS) is simply a sign that there is an imbalance of the muscles that move the eyes. Because this movement is finely coordinated, anything that affects this extremely delicate balance will cause double vision; because true double vision (diplopia) is produced by both eyes, it immediately disappears on closing either eye. Double vision that is present when one eye is closed is extremely rare and usually indicates a functional or psychological disturbance. Diseases other than MS, such as myasthenia gravis or diabetes, also often cause double vision. People also experience double vision when they first start using bifocal lenses.

Numbness and paresthesias (pins and needles or prickly sensations, the sensations of a limb being asleep) are other common symptoms of MS that not infrequently occur in perfectly normal people. Hyperventilation (heavy breathing) is frequently followed by such sensations in normal individuals, and several commonly used medications, especially antidepressant drugs and diuretics ("water pills"), often produce such abnormal sensations as side effects. Interference with blood circulation as well as involvement of the peripheral nerves by conditions such as diabetes, certain medications, a poorly functioning thyroid gland, and others may result in similar complaints. Strokes may also result in numbness that affects an entire side of the body or just one limb. Strokes, however, are more likely to occur in older persons who are past the usual age when MS is first seen. Sensory changes resulting from MS tend to be asymmetrical and often occur quite suddenly. In MS, it is extremely common for a patient to complain of abnormal sensations such as numbness or tingling but without the examining physician being able to detect any objective sensory changes. Unfortunately, this frequently leads to the dismissal of symptoms as being imaginary or unreal.

Incoordination of gait (walking) or poor balance may result from overindulgence in alcohol, or it may be a side effect of some commonly used drugs: tranquilizers, antihistamines, sedatives such as phenobarbital, and anticonvulsant drugs such as phenytoin (Dilantin). Incoordination of the fine movements of the hands is seen less frequently. Trembling of the hands may simply be part of "familial essential tremor," a completely benign condition that begins in youth and is usually found in one parent.

Another source of confusion for both patients and physicians relates to disturbances of urinary bladder function. Frequency, urgency, incontinence (loss of control of the bladder and rarely of the bowel), urinary retention, and nocturia (having to get up in the middle of the night to urinate) may indicate that certain parts of the nervous system are affected by MS. Some of these symptoms may also be caused by a urinary tract or bladder infection, prostate disease, and circulatory problems. Urinary tract infection, which usually causes burning on urination, may be completely painless and thus simulate the symptoms described above.

Weakness of an arm or leg, with or without sensory symptoms (any alteration of sensation, such as numbness or tingling) or incoordination, is frequent in MS but may of course indicate some other disturbance as well. One form of weakness—the rapidly developing, even quite sudden, paralysis of both lower extremities, often associated with loss of sensation in the legs—represents a peculiar manifestation of MS called "transverse myelitis," in which a lesion transects, or "cuts," the spinal cord, disturbing its function. This is usually seen in association with bladder and bowel paralysis.

Certain symptoms are so unusual, they may puzzle both the patient and the physician. A sudden sensation of an electric shock running down the patient's back when the head is flexed suddenly is called "Lhermitte's sign." Occasionally, the same sensation is experienced when bending forward at the waist. It is often erroneously believed that Lhermitte's sign is positive proof of MS, whereas it actually indicates any disturbance very high in the spinal cord. Patients with MS sometimes lose their color vision for a few minutes and are unable to interpret traffic lights correctly at one corner, but by the time they reach the next set of lights, they have recovered the ability to distinguish red from green.

In general, the disease is most difficult to diagnose in its earliest stages. Often, symptoms are considered hysterical (caused by being overly emotional) when they are in fact real. Just as frequently, however, symptoms experienced by some individuals are inconsequential but are interpreted as being symptoms of MS.

THE DIAGNOSTIC PROCESS

Three elements are important to the process of arriving at a diagnosis: (a) the history obtained from the patient, (b) the neurological examination (tests of the nervous system function), and (c) a variety of specialized procedures, which may include examinations of the cerebrospinal fluid (the fluid that courses through the spinal column), certain types of X-rays, and a number of electrical tests (Table 1 outlines the clinical criteria for MS diagnosis).

The problems regarding the history have already been noted. It should be mentioned, however, that another important characteristic of MS, in addition to the presence of multiple, scattered lesions of the nervous system, is that in about two-thirds of MS patients symptoms come and go. These fluctuations are called exacerbations (when the symptoms are present) and remissions (when they are not). These periods are difficult to define, particularly in terms of severity and duration. During remissions, symptoms do not always disappear completely. Often, careful examination reveals that a symptom (for example, loss of sensation or the presence of a prickly sensation) has not

TABLE 1. *Clinical criteria for MS diagnosis*

Onset usually between 10 and 60 years of age.
Symptoms and signs indicating lesions of CNS white matter.
Evidence of two or more lesions on examination.
Objective evidence of CNS disease on neurologic examination.
A course following one of two patterns:
1. Two or more episodes lasting at least 24 hours and occurring at least 1 month apart.
2. A progressive course of signs and symptoms over at least 6 months.

No better explanation for the patient's symptoms and signs.

The revised criteria contain the categories "laboratory-supported clinically definite or clinically probable MS." Included are patients who have evidence of a second lesion only by CT or magnetic resonance imagining or evoked-potential testing, or who have oligoclonal bands in the CSF.

disappeared but, rather, has become less noticeable so that the patient notes a relative improvement. In other situations, the patient has learned to compensate for and ignore what was at first an annoying symptom.

The disease is classified as "possible," "probable," or "definite" based on the physician's ability to demonstrate the presence of more than one lesion in the patient's central nervous system. Until recently, this determination had to be based almost exclusively on information garnered from the history and physical examination. In many cases, that is all that is necessary to establish a diagnosis of definite MS. Today, however, some specialized procedures, particularly measurement of a variety of evoked responses (the recording of electrical activity produced by the brain when it is stimulated by light, sound, or other sensory stimuli), magnetic resonance imaging (MRI), and computer-assisted tomography (CAT scanning, a special kind of X-ray), may confirm the diagnosis when necessary. The term "definite MS" must be viewed with care. There is as yet no absolutely reliable single laboratory procedure that can be performed on the patient, his blood, or his cerebrospinal fluid that by itself establishes the diagnosis of MS.

Many diseases of the central nervous system, at their onset, have exactly the same symptoms and the same abnormalities on both the physical examination and the laboratory tests, but these later prove to be significant for establishing the diagnosis of MS. Therefore, it is often more valuable and certainly less expensive simply to observe the patient over a period of weeks or even months than to perform a series of diagnostic procedures that in the early stage of the disease may only indicate that some central nervous system disorder is present. For this reason, the category of "possible" MS should be avoided.

Neurological Examination

The neurological examination (of the nervous system) is the simplest and often the most convincing way of establishing or confirming the MS diagnosis. The disease affects certain parts of the central nervous system most often, causing characteristic symptoms and signs of abnormal functioning. The symptoms have already been mentioned. However, actual signs of dysfunction cannot always be related to symptoms, as many signs produce no alterations that can be felt or experienced by the patient.

It must also be emphasized that lesions that do not produce any symptom or even signs of malfunction exist in practically every MS patient. It is important for patients to realize this so that they understand that the appearance of a new symptom does not necessarily signify the formation of a new area of involvement. It is difficult to understand how lesions that are discovered at autopsy have not produced symptoms in view of their location and size, but they are seen repeatedly.

When the physician looks into the subject's eyes with his ophthalmoscope, he is examining that portion of the optic nerve that is visible as it penetrates the eyeball. In MS, the optic nerve is often pale, suggesting that it may have been damaged earlier, but the damage did not cause any alteration of visual functions; alternatively, the damage may have produced such a transient visual disturbance that it has been forgotten by the patient. Visual acuity should be tested with an eye chart and using the patient's glasses, if worn, to obtain the best visual acuity (20/20 is normal). Nystagmus is often present. The patient may complain of double vision; the physician will then ask the individual to direct his eyes in various directions and note if both eyes do not move exactly together as they are supposed to do. Sometimes the physician can detect double vision of which the patient has not been aware.

Mild degrees of weakness and incoordination may be detected during the physical examination, as may slight changes in the subject's balance when walking or standing. Examination of the sensory system is quite often disappointing. Despite the fact that the patient clearly describes a pins-and-needles sensation involving an arm or leg, a detailed examination of that limb may reveal no alteration of sensation. This is sometimes true even for such specialized senses as position (the relationship between the patient's body and space) or vibration (the ability to feel the vibration of a tuning apparatus placed on bony protrusions, such as ankles or the fingers). Inequality in the activity of the reflexes on either side or determining that they are overactive is significant. The fact that the big toe goes up rather than down (the Babinski sign) when the outside of the sole of the foot is scratched with a sharp object indicates a disturbance of the major nervous pathways that carry messages from the brain to the muscles, even though the patient may not be aware of such involvement.

The neurological examination is a way of further establishing the fact that a number of separate lesions exist within the central nervous system.

If the abdominal reflexes are absent (the abdominal muscles do not twitch when they are gently stroked with a sharp object), many neurologists consider this an important clue. Unfortunately, such reflexes tend to disappear normally in women who have had several pregnancies and in both men and women who are obese or have had repeated abdominal operations. Many neurological signs are caused by other conditions. Nystagmus, for example, often results from taking commonly prescribed medications, such as diazepam (Valium), sleeping pills, including most barbiturates, and many anticonvulsant drugs. Unequal reflexes (an abnormal finding) may result from injuries to the area where they are being tested, particularly the knees. The physician must be just as careful when interpreting the signs noted in the neurological examination as when he ascribes significance to symptoms and complaints related to him by the patient.

The availability of many laboratory procedures such as neurophysiological testing, examinations of CSF, and CT and MR imaging have greatly extended the physician's diagnostic capability. It should, however, be quite clear that these tests may be useful but that they are not always necessary.

The following is a description of these procedures. None of them is specific for MS, although they are often abnormal in the presence of MS.

Simple Clinical Diagnostic Procedures

An important consideration in MS is the fact that some central nervous system lesions cause no symptoms. There are several techniques that can be used to detect these lesions. These tests are particularly important in patients whose clinical history and physical examination indicate that there is only a single lesion of the central nervous system. In such cases, a search must be made for more lesions in order to confirm the diagnosis of MS.

A simple procedure that is quite useful either in the office or at the bedside is to look for unsuspected unilateral color blindness. Loss of the ability to distinguish colors, most frequently red and green, is very common in MS. It may be the only manifestation of optic neuritis (involvement of the optic nerve), which is a common feature of MS. Few patients are aware of this loss of color vision unless they accidentally shut one eye and discover that the other eye has become colorblind. The doctor can have the patient identify the "hidden" numbers in the Ishihara or AO pseudoisochromatic color plates in order to reveal such color blindness.

Neurophysiological Tests

One of the greatest contributions to the diagnosis of MS has been the development of various techniques for recording and measuring evoked potentials. To explain: When light is flashed into the eyes, or a person is asked to look at a particular light stimulus (such as a black-and-white checkerboard on which the colors are reversed two times per second), electrical activity is produced in a specific part of the brain (the occipital lobe, where all visual impulses are recorded). This electrical activity can be recorded by the electroencephalograph (EEG), a machine that records brain waves. In order for this activity to be separated from the normal activity of the brain, the stimuli are repeated several hundred times, and the resulting brain activity (electrical impulses) is fed into a computer, which converts it into a form that can be interpreted. The resultant activity is what is known as an evoked potential, in this instance, from visual stimuli (visual evoked potential, VEP). Similar information can be obtained by stimulating the ears with clicks (brainstem auditory evoked potential, BAEP) or by stimulating nerves in the arm and in the legs with a mild electric shock (somatosensory evoked potential, SEP) and recording the resulting electrical impulses from the appropriate parts of the brain. Figure 1 shows a subject undergoing visual evoked potential testing.

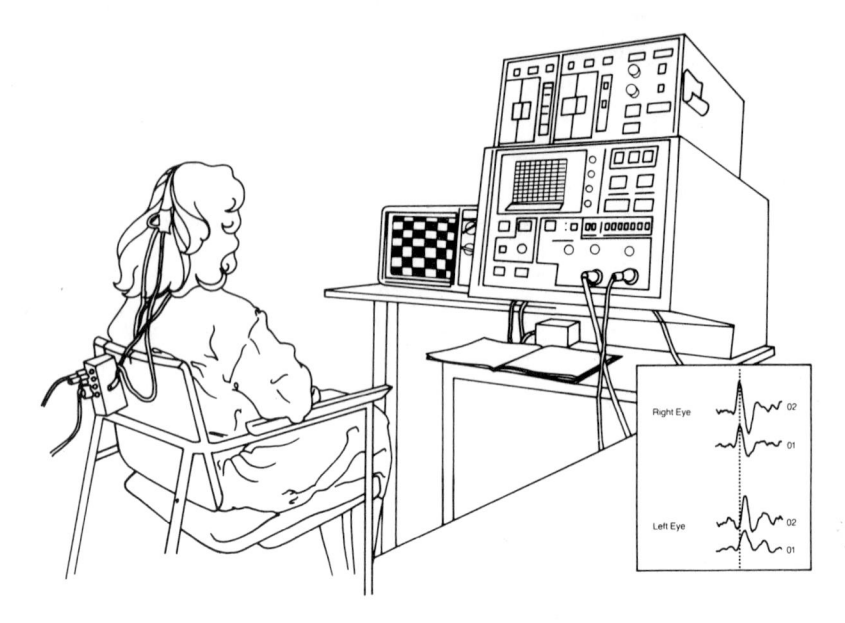

FIG. 1. A patient undergoing visual evoked potential testing.

These procedures are extremely valuable, not only for confirming an already suspected lesion but, more importantly, for demonstrating a completely asymptomatic, unsuspected lesion. They have the advantage of being completely harmless to the patient. Measurement of both the visual and auditory evoked responses is painless, although measuring the somatosensory evoked responses may be uncomfortable because of the strength of the electrical current necessary to stimulate the nerves at the wrist or knee.

The visual evoked responses test is by far the most valuable; this is because it can demonstrate unsuspected lesions of the optic nerves in 75% of patients with MS who have never been aware of any previous alteration of vision. The other two procedures yield fewer positive results but still enough to warrant their use.

There are other more sophisticated but less frequently used tests involving vision. One of the more interesting and still not usually available tests measures contrast sensitivity. It helps to explain the blurring of vision that some MS patients experience. Such blurring results from the eyes' loss of ability to differentiate between various contrasting shades. Another function that is often impaired in MS is the ability to fuse into a single stimulus flickers of light which are separated in time. This is called "impairment of flicker fusion." Only very specialized laboratories are able to carry out these tests.

The EEG (brain wave test) itself, despite the fact that it is frequently ordered in MS patients, is usually of no value. When alterations are present, they are either totally irrelevant to the disease or are completely nonspecific and nondiagnostic. Similarly, electrical examination of nerve and muscle (electromyography, EMG) and nerve conduction velocity testing (NCV) is unwarranted unless either the history or the physical examination suggests involvement of the peripheral nervous system. (The central nervous system—the brain and spinal cord—can be viewed as the main control system of the body. The peripheral nervous system is composed of the nerves branching from the central system that carry messages to and from the central system. The peripheral nervous system is never involved in MS patients.) If there is a peripheral nervous system disturbance, such as a lesion of that system (perhaps as a result of trauma or an alcoholic or diabetic neuropathy), electromyography and/or nerve conduction time testing may be useful.

Imaging Techniques

X-ray examinations of the skull are of no value whatsoever, and radioisotope brain scans are generally of little help. Computer-assisted tomography (CAT scanning, a special X-ray examination) is more valuable in determining the activity of the illness than in establishing the diagnosis, although it may be able to demonstrate the presence of multiple lesions, supporting evidence that may be necessary for the definitive diagnosis of MS or to rule out other causes of symptoms such as tumors or vascular disorders.

The new technique of magnetic resonance imaging is far more sensitive and safer than X-ray procedures. This method does not expose the patient to radiation and requires no injection of radiographic material, although the experience is similar to having a CT scan. The

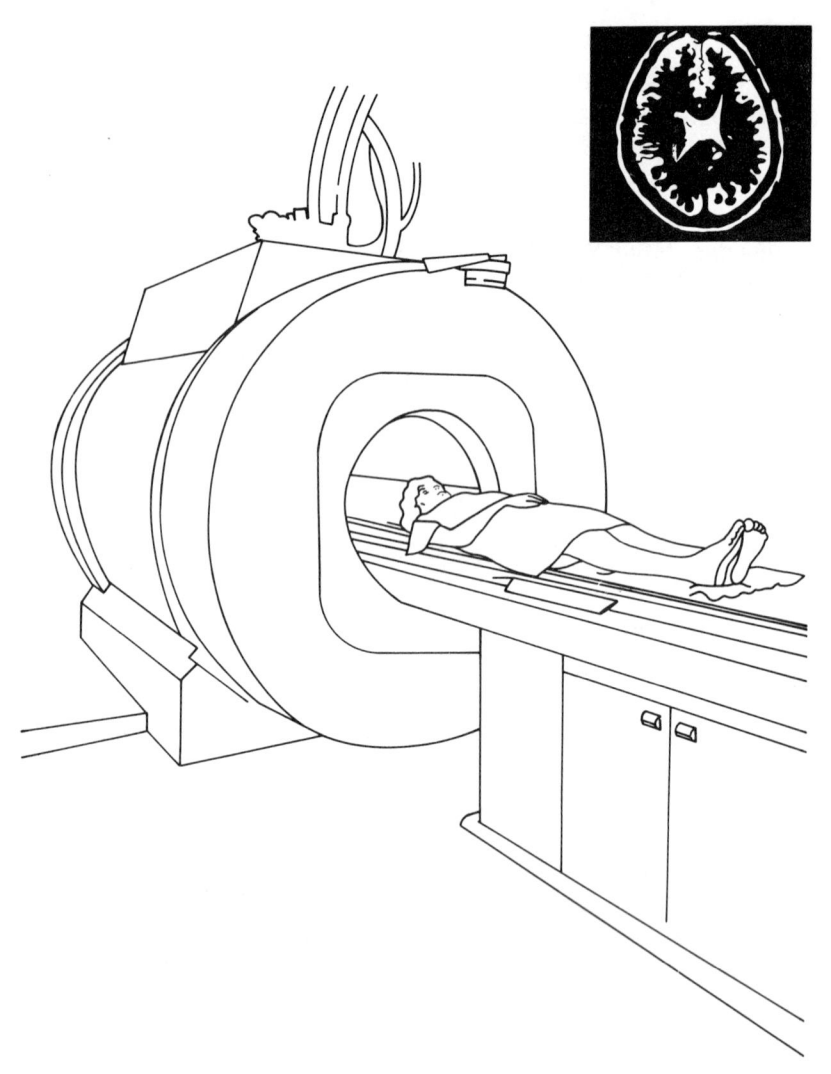

FIG. 2. Magnetic resonance imaging (MRI).

resultant image provides clear evidence of white matter lesions in the brain or spinal cord (Fig. 2).

Myelography is a procedure in which a water-soluble material containing iodine is injected into the spinal canal in order to outline the spinal cord so it can be seen on an X-ray film. It has been said, only half jocularly, that many physicians feel safe in making the diagnosis of MS only after obtaining a negative myelogram. At best, this test is unpleasant, but it also may have serious side effects. It is true that a high cervical (spinal cord) lesion (such as a tumor) may produce symptoms for a time that are like those of MS, including nystagmus. Usually, however, a careful review of the patient's history for visual problems and the demonstration of an abnormality of the visual or brainstem auditory evoked response or MRI abolish the need for a myelogram. The auditory evoked response, the Kimura blink reflex or neuroimaging, and the color vision test are painless and productive and do not require hospital admission.

Cerebrospinal Fluid

For many years, examination of the cerebrospinal fluid was considered absolutely necessary to confirm the diagnosis of MS. Today, in many instances, a spinal tap has become superfluous, since the diagnosis can be confirmed by means of evoked response studies and/or tissue imaging. The abnormalities often found in MS include elevated protein content, increased IgG (an immunoglobulin), and the presence of oligoclonal bands. None of these abnormalities is specific, however.

It was noted some years ago that many patients with MS had abnormal amounts of colloidal gold, and later that MS patients had an increased amount of gamma-globulin in their cerebrospinal fluid. These findings indicated an immunological abnormality, and so the measurement of immunoglobulin G (IgG, a protein fraction of gamma-globulin) became one of the standard diagnostic tests.

An elevation of IgG is not specific for MS; it can be seen in a wide variety of other diseases, and so its elevation alone is not sufficient to establish the diagnosis of MS. In many cases, an incorrect diagnosis of MS has been based almost entirely on this laboratory observation in patients whose history and physical examination barely suggested MS. Furthermore, the reliability of this test varies considerably from hospital to hospital. In some research-oriented institutions, it approaches a reliability of 65 to 70%, but in most others, it is reliable only 40 to 50% of the time. However, it remains a useful confirmatory test in patients whose history and physical examination suggest the diagnosis of MS.

The demonstration of a specific IgG (oligoclonal IgG bands) in cerebrospinal fluid has been reported as being positive in over 90% of patients with MS. Unfortunately, a number of other conditions produce the same abnormality. In performing this test, great attention must be paid to the details of the technique itself, so that its diagnostic value becomes highly questionable in all but a handful of institutions where the test is very carefully controlled. In those places, it is an extraordinarily valuable confirmatory test for MS.

It is also possible now to measure the myelin basic protein (one of the breakdown products of myelin) in cerebrospinal fluid. This particular test is almost useless in making the diagnosis, as the material may be found in the cerebrospinal fluid in any illness in which myelin is destroyed, such as trauma, strokes, or infections. It is also of only minor value for determining the activity of the disease process for the same reason. Neither the elevation of IgG nor the presence of oligoclonal bands in the cerebrospinal fluid gives any indication about the severity of the disease or its degree of activity.

Psychological Examinations

There are many types of psychological tests available today, each of which is designed for specific purposes. Psychological testing, however, rarely provides information of value in the diagnosis but may assist in the management of the MS patient. Textbooks often characterize any mental changes noted in MS as euphoria (a sensation of well-being that persists despite the presence of obvious disabilities). Although euphoria is common, depression is equally so. In addition to mood disturbances, there may be subtle but important intellectual and cognitive deficits. Patients may complain of having difficulty performing their jobs or other intellectual tasks for reasons that cannot be detected by the usual methods of examination. Judiciously chosen psychological tests have revealed a high percentage of cognitive deficits in patients judged by even experienced physicians to be intellectually normal. Furthermore, there appears to be no correlation between the presence of such cognitive deficits and the presence or absence of other functional disability of the motor, sensory, or coordinative systems. Finally, because one of the most common complaints of MS patients is lack of energy, psychological evaluation may be useful in differentiating this complaint from depression. The complaint of fatigability is often (erroneously) thought to be caused by depression in MS patients: the fatigue is real, although it is extremely difficult to ascribe it to weakness, stiffness, or any other physical causes.

Laboratory Examinations

Blood Tests

There are no abnormalities of the red blood cells, white blood cells, or platelets (cells involved in the clotting process) or of the chemical constituents of blood that provide any diagnostic clues in MS.

Immunological Tests

Many tests of immunological function (the body's system of defense against infection and other foreign substances) have been developed. None has any value in the diagnosis of MS at this time. Most immunological tests are not only highly specialized and not generally available, but their results vary considerably from one laboratory to the other, and their significance remains unclear.

Genetic Tests

The "histocompatibility system" consists of genetic material on a particular chromosome that controls the ability of a person to accept or reject tissue transplants (such as kidney). Principally in Scandinavia and the United States, where large groups of MS patients have been studied, it has been demonstrated that specific types of this genetic material are present in a significant number of MS patients. From these studies has come the interesting suggestion that certain genetic factors may predispose individuals to acquire MS. Studies have also been carried out in families in which more than one blood relative was affected by the disease. These studies have not provided any basis for the hope that examining the histocompatibility system in MS patients might reveal this predisposition. In one study, the genetic characteristics of two siblings with MS in the same family were shown to be completely different, whereas in other families, patients with MS and normal siblings shared identical genetic factors. Some medical centers have tried to use the information derived from such studies to help diagnose MS in individuals, but to no avail.

DIAGNOSIS OF AN EXACERBATION

Diagnosing a return of the symptoms of MS (that is, an exacerbation of the disease) remains critical to the management of a diagnosed patient. There are no definite clinical criteria by which we can judge that the disease process has been activated. Obviously, such a determination is of the utmost importance in instituting treatment and evaluating if it is effective.

New symptoms occur in only about one-fifth of patients with exacerbation of their disease. In other words, in four of five patients, symptoms noted when the disease flares are simply a recurrence of those experienced before. Because we now know that lesions do exist that never cause symptoms, new symptoms cannot necessarily be interpreted as evidence of the formation of new lesions; in fact, they may stem from lesions that have been "silent" up to now. The same thing is true of new signs.

In addition to the fact that a temperature elevation produces symptoms, other physiological disturbances (such as alterations in water and salt metabolism caused, for example, by vomiting and diarrhea) may similarly lead to the appearance of symptoms. The most common cause of exacerbation of symptoms is elevated temperature because of a body infection, usually of the bladder. These are often transient and may be called "pseudoexacerbations." Fatigue and psychological stress may play a role in the increased physical impairment. Because of this, hospitalization or even simple bed rest, and thus removal from the daily stress of work and home, may lead to the disappearance of often serious symptoms.

It bears repeating that exacerbations do not necessarily represent an aggravation of the disease. The rate of activity of the disease cannot be determined on the basis of clinical symptoms. In the same way, "improvement" brought about by certain forms of treatment may be caused more by the enthusiasm of the dedicated investigator than by the treatment itself.

INFORMING THE PATIENT

Patients and their immediate families have every right to be told the diagnosis, especially the degree of certainty with which it has been established. The physician should be the one to relate this information, but physicians are often loath to do this, as they fear it will produce severe depression. In fact, a forthright discussion will enhance the trust necessary to the physician–patient relationship. Moreover, being told the name of the illness and the nature of its course will aid in more rapid adjustment and subsequent rehabilitation. Therefore, the use of such terms as "demyelinating disease," "inflammation of the white matter," or even "possible" MS are counterproductive and will needlessly extend the period of anxiety for the patient.

A patient should be assured that, contrary to popular belief, MS does not carry a uniformly poor prognosis. It should be pointed out that (a) many MS patients have the disease in so mild a form that they never suffer any kind of disability because of it; (b) in others, the dysfunction is mild and temporary; (c) the disease seems to be arrested or burned out in many patients; and (D) it is a minority of MS patients who end up bedridden. A patient should be told not only to avoid heat but also how to take care of minor infections and prevent urinary tract infections. Such general supportive measures can be of great help in improving long-term prognosis.

Patients with MS tend, as do others with slowly progressive or chronic illnesses, to seek other opinions and to search for new forms of treatment. If a patient is reluctant to accept the diagnosis of MS, it may be best to get a second opinion as quickly as possible from another competent neurologist. All treatments should be carefully explained and discussed with the patient and family. Reassurance, sound information, and compassion must always be available for the MS patient.

CONCLUSION

It is often difficult to make a diagnosis of MS in its early stages. If the disease progresses, this becomes easy. The diagnosis is based on the demonstration—by the history, physical examination, and carefully chosen diagnostic procedures—that there are multiple lesions scattered throughout the white matter of the central nervous system. For many patients, laboratory procedures are not necessary but may be useful in confirming the clinical impression. Usually, adequate confirmation can be obtained by the noninvasive, relatively inexpensive, simple procedure of measuring visual or other types of evoked responses. Magnetic resonance imaging is a promising new technique that appears to be more sensitive than the CAT scan, which has limited usefulness in diagnosing this illness. Examination of the cerebrospinal fluid has been largely supplanted by other tests.

There is a natural tendency on the part of physicians to play it safe by ordering many tests that may in some way or another support the diagnosis. Engaging in such a diagnostic cascade, unfortunately at times demanded by the patient, is not only unwarranted but becomes extremely expensive and unpleasant and is also potentially harmful.

Multiple Sclerosis: A Guide for Patients and Their Families, Second Edition, edited by L. C. Scheinberg and N. J. Holland. Raven Press © 1987.

5

Signs and Symptoms of Multiple Sclerosis

Labe C. Scheinberg and Charles R. Smith

Multiple sclerosis is the most common of the neurological diseases characterized by demyelination of the brain and spinal cord. Many individuals, including some health care professionals, mistakenly think that once a diagnosis of MS is made, a wheelchair-bound existence will inevitably follow. Although it is a chronic disease, it is not necessarily progressive.

This chapter outlines the most common signs and symptoms of the MS patient, describes the possible courses of the disease, and discusses what predictions can be made about the eventual outcome.

PREVALENCE AND INCIDENCE

In the United States, about 58 persons per 100,000 population—the prevalence—carry a diagnosis of MS, yielding a population of about 123,000. However, the actual number may be much higher. There are several reasons for this; two are listed here. First, many people with tingling in the limbs or blurring of vision, minor neurological symptoms of MS, may ignore these or attribute them to another illness such as a viral infection, neuritis, or arthritis. Second, many physicians are simply reluctant to diagnose MS. It is interesting that the signs of MS are occasionally seen at autopsy in patients dying of other causes, though review of their medical records reveals no documentation of complaints or findings indicating nervous system disease.

Just as MS tends to occur more often in temporate and colder regions of the world, it also occurs more commonly in the northern half of the United States. Above the 37th parallel, the chance of getting MS—the incidence—is almost twice that below. The overall incidence of MS in the United States is 4.2 persons per 100,000, or 8,800 new cases per year.

Multiple sclerosis is mainly a disease of white women. The female-to-male ratio is more than 2 to 1. The white-to-nonwhite ratio is about 2 to 1. The disease is most common in the 20- to 60-year age group with a peak age of onset around 33 years. There are, however, many who experience their first symptoms after the age of 60, and the disease has even been seen in children.

SIGNS AND SYMPTOMS

The signs and symptoms of MS can be called primary, secondary, or tertiary. Primary symptoms are the result of an area of demyelination, also called a plaque, and include symptoms such as weakness, numbness, urinary incontinence, visual disturbance, and fatigue. Secondary symptoms are complications that result from the primary ones, including urinary bladder infection and pressure sores. Tertiary symptoms include the emotional, social, and vocational impact of the disease on the patient, family, and community.

Table 1 lists in order of frequency of occurrence the primary symptoms experienced during the first attack of MS. Table 2 lists the likelihood of a symptom being experienced during the course of MS.

TABLE 1. *Frequency of initial symptoms*

Symptom	Incidence
Sensory disturbance of limbs	33%
Disturbance of gait and balance	18%
Visual loss in one eye	17%
Double vision	13%
Progressive weakness	10%
Acute myelitis syndrome	6%
Sensory disturbance of face	3%
Lhermitte's symptom	3%
Pain	2%

TABLE 2. *Frequency of symptoms during course of illness*

Symptom	Incidence
Balance abnormalities	78%
Impaired sensation	71%
Fatigue	65%
Paraparesis	62%
Urinary disturbance	62%
Sexual disturbance	60%
Visual loss in one eye	55%
Weakness of one limb	52%
Incoordination of limbs	45%
Double vision	43%
Abnormal sensory experiences	40%
Pain	25%
Facial paralysis	15%
Epilepsy	5%
Hearing loss	4%
Facial pain (tic douloureux)	2%

Primary Symptoms

Multiple sclerosis is largely a disorder of walking (gait) and bowel and bladder (sphincter) function. Plaques of demyelination can arise in any part of the brain or spinal cord that is the central nervous system. Because a lot of myelin or white matter is needed for the control of gait and sphincter function, symptoms referrable to these are the most frequent.

Abnormal gait may result from weakness of the legs, stiffness (spasticity), imbalance, or any combination of these. Spasticity and weakness frequently result when the spinal cord is involved. An early symptom of spasticity is stiffness of the legs described as "heaviness," "dragging," or "easily fatigued." Patients may say that it is difficult to walk over rough surfaces such as carpets and unpaved walkways. In the earliest phases of spasticity, patients say that they can not walk quickly or run. There is increasing difficulty in climbing stairs and in dealing with roadside curbs. Toes of shoes may wear out, primarily along the instep. All these problems may worsen when weakness of the legs is also present. These symptoms may seem to involve only one leg, but physical examination usually shows involvement of both.

Patients with spasticity frequently experience spasms in their lower limbs. These may occur spontaneously or as a result of stimulation, i.e., turning in bed at night. This is from dragging the feet across the bed sheets. These spasms can be painful and are similar to a "charley horse" if the calf is affected. Frequency of such spasms might increase when there is a bladder infection, constipation, or when there are painful foot ailments such as ingrown toenails. Patients may then mistakenly feel that they are experiencing an exacerbation of their disease when in fact the spasms are related to the irritating stimulus. Accordingly, these "worsenings" are called pseudoexacerbations. With spasticity, the patient often notices shaking or jerking of the leg when the toe is placed on the floor and the knee is slightly bent. This sign of spasticity is called clonus.

If the arms are weak or spastic, patients complain that they have problems doing anything requiring fine finger movements. Doing up buttons, tying shoelaces, and writing may be particularly difficult.

Problems with coordination and balance may be very disabling. *Ataxia* is a frequent symptom characterized by the patient's inability to balance while walking. This necessitates walking with the feet spread more widely apart than normal, improving the center of gravity. Plaques in part of the brain known as the cerebellum are usually responsible.

Tremor of the limbs and of the head and trunk are also signs that the cerebellum is affected. With hand tremor, the patient often notes that this symptom worsens when attempting to exercise precise control of the fingers (intention tremor). This frustrating experience may make writing, eating, and dressing nearly impossible.

Other cerebellar signs include incoordination of speech and disturbance of eye movement. Many people with cerebellar plaques may speak indistinctly, as if drunk, or may exhibit nystagmus, oscillations of the eyes in certain positions. This is usually only noticed by the physician during examination. However, some types of nystagmus give rise to symptoms: objects may seem to shimmer or jump when the patient tries to focus on them, a condition called oscillopsia.

Complaints of *abnormal sensation* like "tingling," "pins and nee-

SIGNS AND SYMPTOMS

dles," or "tight bands" are very common. Some patients have painful sensations, which can be either aching or sharp and shooting. These sensory problems can occur in any part of the body and are most frequent in the legs and trunk. Sometimes they are confused with other diseases such as carpal tunnel syndrome when aching pain occurs in the hand, sciatica when pain goes down the back of the leg, and tic douloureux, a shooting pain that occurs in otherwise healthy older people, when pain involves the face. Many exhibit sensory abnormalities on examination, most frequently a reduction of vibration sense in the legs, determined by testing with the tuning fork.

A majority of patients complain of *problems with bladder and bowel function,* bladder symptoms being the most troublesome. The most frequent bladder symptoms are a sense of urgency, frequency of urination occurring both day and night, and incontinence. Others complain of inability to empty the bladder, noting hesitancy when starting urination, a weak stream, or interruption of the urinary stream while voiding. Because some bladder problems can lead to complications, a worsening of a patient's complaints may indicate infection and not a worsening of MS. Again, this is a pseudoexacerbation. For this reason, many physicians check the urine for infection when such changes are reported.

Equally common are bowel function problems, the major complaint being constipation. Urgency or incontinence is also common.

Sexual problems are regularly reported. Common are failure to achieve erection or impotence in males and failure to achieve orgasm or climax in females. Impotence may not be secondary to neurological lesions but may in part reflect psychological reactions to the primary disease. Failure to climax is usually a result of decreased sensation in the genital area.

Complaints of *reduced vision* are frequent in MS, specifically, blurring and sometimes loss of vision in one eye. This is called optic neuritis and is caused by a plaque of demyelination affecting the optic nerve. Persistent severe loss of vision is uncommon, though during the first few days there may be discomfort in the eye and profound visual loss. Occasionally after an attack of optic neuritis, the physician can see the actual effects of the attack of the optic nerve, using an ophthalmoscope. The optic nerve head or disk looks pale. Another visual complaint is diplopia or double vision, only apparent when looking in specific directions.

Impairment of intellect is uncommon in MS but may be seen in patients who have advanced disease. Contrary to popular opinion, inappropriate elation or euphoria is much less common than depression.

The majority of patients complain of *abnormal fatigability*. It is a major problem in a third of patients, who describe it as a "washed-out," "exhausted," or "lacking in energy" sensation, usually worse in the mid- to late afternoon. The cause of this is unknown, but since it seems to worsen with warm and humid weather, it may be secondary to changes in body temperature. Normally, body temperature is highest in the late afternoon and lowest early in the morning.

Dizziness or vertigo is often reported, a symptom in which there may be a sensation of spinning or turning, sometimes associated with nausea or vomiting. Such a symptom is usually short-lived.

Significant *hearing loss* is uncommon in MS and is usually detected only with quantitative hearing tests.

Secondary Symptoms

Secondary problems are complications of the neurological ones and a source of much suffering. They are frequently responsible for the shortened life span of those who die prematurely from the disease, and the MS caregiver must educate both patient and family on their prevention.

Fibrous contractures can result when severe spasticity is unrelieved by medication or other treatments. This permanent shortening of overactive muscles can cause abnormal limb postures, making it impossible for the patient to sit or lie down properly. Joints might become fused as a result of these abnormal postures, possibly leading to another problem, namely, pressure sores.

Pressure sores, also called bed sores or decubitus ulcers, happen when excessive pressure on the skin and tissues beneath prevents the flow of blood. They tend to occur over bony prominences or where there is sustained excessive pressure, commonly on the buttocks, thighs, and heels. Patients with significant paralysis or loss of sensation must

SIGNS AND SYMPTOMS

be moved periodically to relieve these effects of pressure. Other factors may enhance the development of pressure sores, such as improper wheelchair posture, friction from being dragged across bedsheets, and excessive moisture from incontinence of urine. Pressure sores are always infected and can cause deeper infection involving nearby bone (osteomyelitis) or may track into nearby joints (pyarthrosis).

Urinary tract infection (UTI) is another frequent complication of MS and is caused by incomplete emptying of the bladder. Bladder infections can cause spread of infection to the kidneys (pyelonephritis) and kidney or bladder stones.

Occasionally, patients develop *swallowing problems*. They may develop pneumonia if the contents of the mouth, be it saliva or ingested foods or liquids, fall into the respiratory tract. For this reason, patients with swallowing problems should be evaluated by a speech therapist, who identifies those most at risk for such complications and who recommends the best treatment.

Tertiary Symptoms

As in any chronic, unpredictable illness, there are frequently tertiary symptoms in the psychosocial and vocational areas. To cope with the stress of the illness, an MS patient must mobilize support from many sources. Sources may be external—family, friends, colleagues, and medical personnel—or internal—the individual's own sense of health, attitudes, and coping strategies learned throughout life. One role of the physician is to identify persons with insufficient or defective support systems in order to initiate contacts with available resources, i.e., psychological and family counseling, vocational rehabilitation, and occupational therapy. With this help, the patient's own defenses can be maximized.

COURSE OF THE DISEASE

Because the course of MS is variable, one cannot easily predict the outcome in any individual case. However, MS is rarely fatal. The reduction in life span from that predicted is only in the range of

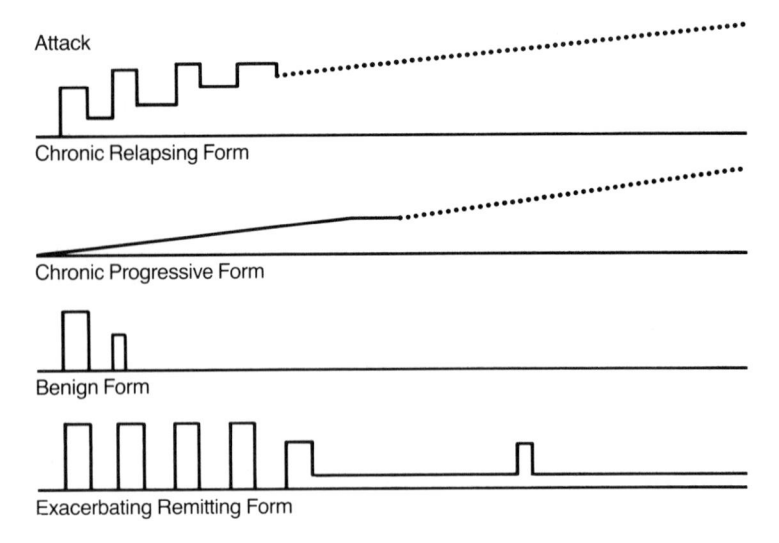

FIG.1 Possible courses of MS.

10% to 15%. Many who do die prematurely die as a result of complications that are often preventable.

Multiple sclerosis tends to adopt certain patterns and may be divided into four basic types: benign, relapsing/remitting, relapsing/progressive, and progressive (Fig. 1). A relapse or exacerbation is the sudden or relatively sudden onset of new symptoms that last for at least one day. A remission refers to improvement in neurological symptoms lasting at least one month to be significant. The improvement may be complete or partial.

The benign type is seen in at least 20% of patients. These patients have few attacks and complete or nearly complete remissions. Their symptoms tend to be primarily sensory or visual. Such persons experience no restrictions in their daily activities and remain fully employed.

The relapsing/remitting type is similar to the benign course except that exacerbations may include episodes of weakness, imbalance, or disturbed bladder function, to name but a few. Like the benign type, there tends to be complete or nearly complete recovery between attacks. After many years of illness, these patients have only mild restrictions, if any, on daily activities. They account for about 25% of patients.

The relapsing/progressive type is also characterized by clearcut attacks, but recovery from such episodes is incomplete. These persons may eventually have moderate to severe disability, with significant restrictions in their activities. About 40% of patients are in this category.

Finally, there are patients who never experience clear exacerbations but who experience instead a slowly progressive disease in which remissions do not occur. In some of these patients, severe disability may be present after only a few years of illness. Only about 15% of patients are in this category.

OUTCOME

Although it is impossible to predict accurately the course a patient will follow, some symptoms seem to be of predictive value. Early onset of illness, before the age of 35, tends to have a better prognosis than disease of later onset. Acute onset of symptoms over days is a much more favorable sign than is gradual onset over weeks or months. Complete remission from the initial attack is also characteristically favorable. When symptoms are primarily of a sensory type, including numbness, tingling or tightness, or optic neuritis, outcome is generally favorable. Early onset of weakness, spasticity, or incoordination, especially affecting gait, is generally a poor prognostic sign. After the first 5 years, one can better predict what the course will be. However, a previously benign course or relapsing/remitting course may evolve into a relapsing/progressive or slowly progressive course. Once a course has become progressive, reversion to a remitting one is not likely.

There has been much speculation over the years about the cause of a new attack. The most frequent factors cited by patients and families are emotional stress and psychological trauma. It is difficult to prove or disprove the role of emotions in the precipitation of attacks or in progression. The sudden appearance of new symptoms may itself cause that emotional distress. To date, studies of this question have revealed only conflicting results. There is still no evidence that pregnancy, physical stress, or psychological trauma can precipitate an MS attack or turn a previously mild course into a severe one.

6

Drug Therapy

Labe C. Scheinberg and Barbara S. Giesser

The goals of therapy of any disease are to prevent the initial occurrence (prophylactic treatment), to arrest the progress of the disease and prevent future attacks (curative treatment), to repair the damaged tissues and restore normal function (restorative treatment), to treat symptoms and prevent and relieve complications (symptomatic treatment), and to help the patient to adjust to the disability and achieve as much function as possible with the remaining normal tissues or parts (rehabilitative treatment).

The cause of MS is not known. Moreover, one can only conjecture about the mechanism of tissue damage that produces the impairment. Finally, it is the nature of the tissues of the central nervous system to regenerate poorly, if at all, after severe damage. Considering these factors, the treatment of MS is very frustrating and disappointing.

At present there is little or probably no treatment that will prevent the initial or future attacks of MS. Although there is excellent prophylactic treatment in many infectious diseases (for example, poliomyelitis, smallpox, measles), there is nothing available for MS because no virus or other infectious agent has been identified. Recently MS was reported theoretically to be related to distemper in dogs, and it has been suggested that eradication of distemper by immunizing dogs would reduce or eliminate MS. However, this is controversial and unproved. It also does little or nothing to help MS patients who already have significant damage and disability.

There are no known curative therapies that will arrest the course of MS or even alter the natural history of attacks and remissions or halt progression. Many approaches have been employed over the last century, and many new methods of treatment are undergoing clinical testing, but it is highly debatable if anything will significantly change the pattern of the disease at this time. It has been reported that certain hormones [for example, cortisone or adrenocorticotropic hormone (ACTH or corticotropin)] shorten an individual attack but do not prevent future attacks and probably have little or no effect on the long-term functioning of the patient. Other drugs and treatments have produced less evidence of benefits, and many reported "cures" or ameliorations are probably coincidental to the natural fluctuations of the disease.

Many symptoms and signs do clear partially, or even completely, following an attack. It is believed that these partial or complete remissions are caused by the clearing of inflammation and edema in the acute lesions. In large and more severe lesions, the myelin at the center of the lesion, or plaque, may be severely damaged, and so only partial or possibly no remission occurs. With subsequent attacks, the lesions, or plaques, enlarge, and the deficit increases, which explains why early in the course of MS many treatments are effective and later most are ineffective.

Once there is a large plaque or lesion in the central myelin with sclerosis (scarring), one must hope that there is some treatment that will restore or repair the damaged myelin and/or improve nerve conduction through the damaged area. Unfortunately, at present there is no restorative therapy that will repair the damage or improve conduction in the region of the plaque.

Today symptomatic and rehabilitative therapy are the most effective approaches available. One may use drugs effectively to relieve certain symptoms (such as spasticity or pain) that are a direct result of the plaques (lesions) in the myelin of the central nervous system. Symptoms such as weakness, spasticity, incoordination, pain, numbness, urinary urgency, incontinence, retention, blurred vision, and others are "primary symptoms" that are related to plaques in specific locations. Other symptoms, such as urinary tract infections (cystitis), bed sores (decubiti), and contractures of joints, are a result of the primary symptoms and should be called "secondary symptoms." These are generally responsive to drug, surgical, or physical therapies and are discussed in detail later. Finally, there are symptoms and other developments that are a result of the primary and secondary symptoms; these should be called "tertiary symptoms" and include such problems as depression, marital problems, loss of employment, etc. These tertiary symptoms or problems are often amenable to psychosocial interventions such as counseling and job modification. These approaches are discussed extensively in later chapters.

Treatment can be divided into four general categories:

1. Pharmacological—use of drugs (chemicals, biological, etc.).
2. Surgical—use of such surgical measures as cutting nerves or tendons, skin grafts, etc.
3. Physical—use of exercises, massage, stretching, heat, cold, or electrical stimulation.
4. Psychological—use of counseling or other psychiatric treatment.

An excellent reference to most of the therapies currently being employed is the book *Therapeutic Claims in Multiple Sclerosis,* published under the auspices of the International Federation of Multiple Sclerosis Society, 205 East 42nd Street, New York, NY 10017. The book reviews about 120 treatments, giving the rationales, benefits, and risks for each. It has been updated as new treatments are developed or the use of experimental ones is proved or disproved. This book is highly recommended and will even counter the sometimes insistent advice of well-meaning family and friends.

GENERAL GUIDELINES IN MANAGEMENT

It is important to state some general guidelines in the management prior to discussion of specific treatments. These have been learned by experience with large numbers of patients and families.

The patient and significant others should be informed of the diagnosis when the neurologist or other competent physician is certain of it. The diagnosis should be "multiple sclerosis," a term most people know, and not such terms as "demyelinating disease," "chronic virus infections of the nervous system," "allergy of the nervous system," "encephalomyelitis," etc.

When patients are not informed at the time the diagnosis is established but learn of it later, they may become angry at the initial physician and not trust him. Often patients are relieved to learn the diagnosis because they had suspected a more serious condition or believed that they had a psychological disorder. Almost all patients can accept the diagnosis and cope with it. It is essential to reveal the diagnosis so that patients and families can plan for the future, avail themselves of the various services and benefits that are available to MS patients, and embark on a sound therapeutic regimen. The diagnosis should be discussed fully along with a presentation of current knowledge of the disease. It should not be unduly optimistic or pessimistic, as the future course cannot be predicted.

The patient should be given a return appointment and not told, "There's no cure, so just go home and learn to live with it." The frequency of return visits depends on the severity, rate of progression, complications, and other factors. The return visits are useful for detecting and treating new findings of MS and complications, for counseling the patient and family, and for discussing new developments in treatment and research.

The patient should be managed when necessary by a team of health professionals consisting of neurologists, physiatrist, psychiatrist, urologist, internists, nurses, physical therapists, occupational therapists, social workers, rehabilitation counselors, and psychologists. Few diseases have as many varied long-term ramifications, and few require the services of so many professionals at some time or other during their course. Few solo practitioners are prepared to deal with so complex a disease during its long course. Not all cases require these services, but patients and families should be aware of the possibilities should the need ever arise.

The patient should participate actively in his management. This disease, as do so many others, makes the patient feel that he or she has lost control, and so he should be encouraged to participate in the adjustment of certain drugs, management of the bladder, rehabilitation, diet, and physical therapy. Most therapeutic decisions are somewhat empirical, and the patient can effectively participate. When the patient does not follow instructions or embarks on a treatment course not

DRUG THERAPY

recommended by the physician, later recriminations should be avoided. With the exception of surgery, unproved treatments often do not cause the disease to worsen but may incur unnecessary expense and, later, disappointment.

The patient should fully discuss any new treatments and be warned about unwarranted optimism. Over the decades most "cures" have not withstood the test of time and have often benefited only the therapists.

In this presentation of drug management, only those agents that we generally employ are discussed. There are many schedules for any drug, but only those we have found to be easily followed and of benefit are presented. Occasionally some other drugs or routes of administration are discussed briefly, as these may be used by other physicians.

DRUG THERAPY OF PRIMARY SYMPTOMS

The major primary symptoms of MS are motor disabilities (weakness, stiffness or spasticity, incoordination, loss of balance, gait difficulties, and tremors). Weakness and other motor symptoms, if seen as part of an acute attack, may respond to short-term antiinflammatory agents such as ACTH (adrenocorticotropic hormone or corticotropin), adrenal corticosteroids, and synthetic glucocorticoids (prednisone). These drugs are administered for brief periods, almost never more than 1 month at a time. Long-term or chronic use is not recommended. The drug may be taken again for brief periods if there is a recurrence or a new attack, but the effect is often less in each subsequent bout. Our method is to give either ACTH or prednisone in the following manner (see Table 1), as we have found it to be simpler, to be less costly, and to have fewer side effects while offering as great a benefit as other methods. Moreover, these methods generally do not require hospital care, and injections may be given by a visiting nurse or other competent individual.

Prednisone, taken on alternate days for 1 month, seems to be as effective as other regimens, and the schedule is simple with few complications. Prednisone, adrenal corticosteroids, and synthetic glucocorticoids may be taken by other routes (intravenous, intramuscular, or

TABLE 1. *Types of steroid regimes*

Steroid	Route	Dose/duration
ACTH	I.M.	80 u/day for 5 days, then 40 u/day for 5 days
Prednisone	Oral	10 mg four times daily on alternate days for one month
Dexamethasone	Oral	16 mg/day for 4 days, 12 mg/day for 3 days, 8 mg/day for 2 days, 4 mg/day for 1 day
Solu-Medrol	I.V.	2 g/day for 2 days, 1 g/day for 2 days, 500 mg/day for 2 days, 250 mg/day for 2 days

intraspinal/intrathecal). Some studies suggest that "pulse" therapy, i.e., high doses of steroids given intravenously for several days and then rapidly tapered and stopped, is effective for treating acute exacerbations. There is no evidence that intraspinal injections of steroids are any more effective than oral, intravenous, or intramuscular routes in treating acute attacks, and the former may be more hazardous and costly.

On an outpatient basis, ACTH may be given intramuscularly. This seems to be as effective as when it is given by the intravenous route, does not require hospitalization or confinement to bed for any period, and is less expensive without risk of hospital-acquired complications.

Again, there is little proof that ACTH and adrenal corticosteroids are very effective except for short-term use to reduce the severity of individual acute attacks. In fact, adrenal corticosteroids have never been tested properly for this disease, and their use has been based on the results of ACTH studies. It has even been stated that if two large groups of MS patients were using ACTH and adrenal corticosteroids for acute attacks (in one group) or nothing (in the other group), the final disability in the two groups would be identical after 10 to 20 years. There is certainly no basis for long-term chronic use of either of these agents.

The complications of therapy with these agents are minimal with short-term use. They include transiently generalized puffiness, weight gain, psychosis (infrequent), peptic ulcer with bleeding, general infections, and acne. With long-term daily therapy, there is in addition the risk of abnormalities in blood levels of sodium and potassium, bone softening with fractures, cataracts, hypertension, diabetes, and adrenal exhaustion.

In conclusion, short-term therapy with ACTH or adrenal corticosteroids carries little risk and seems to be of value in reducing the severity of an individual bout, whereas long-term use does not appear to alter the course and is hazardous. Steroids may be given as summarized in Table 1.

Spasticity is a motor symptom that can be disabling and painful. It may cause difficulty in walking, restrict the range of motion of the extremities, and result in painful muscle spasms. If not properly managed it may result in urinary complications, contractures of the joints, and eventually pressure sores (decubitus ulcers). Three agents have been recommended for controlling spasticity: baclofen (Lioresal), diazepam (Valium), and dantrolene sodium (Dantrium). We employ only baclofen. Diazepam seems to be less effective, produces excessive sedation, and even causes psychic and physical dependence; and dantrolene sodium produces nausea, diarrhea, and carries a long-term risk of liver damage and pleural effusions (fluid collection in the chest). A new antispasticity agent, tizanidine, has been used widely in Europe and is now being tested in the United States. It appears to be as safe and effective as Lioresal.

The recommended dose of baclofen is from 15 mg (1½ tablets) daily to 80 mg (eight tablets) daily given in three or four doses. Occasionally a higher dose must be taken to alleviate severe spasticity; this may be as much as 200 mg a day, even though the Federal Drug Administration (FDA) recommends a maximum of 80 mg a day. Initially, some patients complain of drowsiness, but this is transitory. Others complain of loss of appetite and nausea, both of which can be avoided by taking the drug after meals. More important, many patients report increased sensation of weakness of the legs and greater gait difficulties with this drug. This is related to the reduction of spasticity, making the weakness already present more apparent. Because the dividing line between spasticity and weakness is indistinct, we often advise patients to adjust the dose themselves from time to time. If one takes too much, the legs are excessively flaccid or "rubbery," and the patient feels that his legs are weaker and no longer support him; the dose should be reduced. A return to the previous level of spasticity occurs within hours after changing the dose. If one takes an insufficient dose, the legs feel too spastic or "tight," and the dose should be increased.

Withdrawal from the drug should be done gradually over a few days, because transient seizures and hallucinations have been reported, although rarely.

Tremor, loss of coordination, ataxia, and loss of balance with gait difficulties are troublesome and disabling symptoms and unfortunately are resistant to any known drugs. Some have tried propranolol (Inderal) to relieve tremor, but we have found this agent to have no benefit even at very high dosage. Propranolol may produce too great a drop in blood pressure and can aggravate asthma.

Some patients have appeared to benefit from clonazepam (Clonopin). This drug has reduced tremor and jumping of the eyes (opsoclonus) in approximately 50% of patients in our experience. The drug is generally well tolerated, with sedation being the major side effect. Some doctors have tried isoniazid (INH) for treatment of tremor. We have not found this drug to be effective, and recent studies do not show proven benefit.

Speech disorders, such as slurring, scanning, or unintelligible speech, another motor symptom, do not respond to any currently available drug. Fortunately, they are rarely disabling.

Sensory symptoms (such as numbness, tingling, pins and needles, and pain) are common but usually not disabling or permanent. When the pain is stabbing or lancinating in quality, it should be treated with carbamazepine (Tegretol). Phenytoin (Dilantin) and amitriptyline (Elavil and others) are often useful for painful numbness, burning, or tingling. This is usually effective with minimal side effects (drowsiness, loss of appetite, and nausea). The patients should be followed regularly by their physician, who should closely monitor the effects of the drug. Doses and side effects are summarized in Table 2.

TABLE 2. *Treatment of sensory symptoms*

Drug	Symptoms	Dose (mg/day)	Tablet size (mg)	Side effects
Elavil (amitriptyline)	Burning Pins and needles	25–150	25, 50	Dry mouth, drowsiness, blurred vision, urinary retention
Dilantin (phenytoin)	Burning	300	100	Drowsiness, nausea, gum irritation
Tegretol (carbamazepine)	Trigeminal neuralgia Radicular pain	200–1,600	200	Drowsiness, loss of balance, nausea, urinary retention
Nardil (phenelezine sulfate)	Burning or stabbing pain	45–60	15	Dry mouth, low blood pressure (may produce dangerous hypertension if dietary restrictions are not followed)

Amitriptyline (Elavil) has also been shown to be effective in some patients who have "emotional incontinence" or uncontrollable inappropriate laughing or crying.

Other sensory symptoms (such as visual symptoms) also do not cause significant disability, and we rarely use any drugs in these cases. Occasionally, one may employ ACTH or adrenal corticosteroids for severe visual symptoms caused by inflammation of the optic nerve, especially if there is pain in the eye. These symptoms are usually transient and in most cases clear spontaneously within 2 to 3 months or less. Vertigo is usually transitory and may be treated with meclazine hydrochloride (Antivert or Bonine).

Many patients with MS find that they are incapacitated by fatigue even if they are not severely physically disabled. Amantidine (Symmetrel) has been reported to be effective in alleviating this fatigue in some patients. We have found that pemoline (Cylert) is also effective in treating fatigue. It is most effective when taken a few hours before the onset of fatigue. Side effects include insomnia and potential for dependency.

Urinary symptoms are common, and it is important to manage them carefully. One of the major approaches to this is drug therapy in conjunction with other measures (Chapter 11).

The use of certain drugs to control muscle contractions of the urinary bladder is important when the patient complains of primary urinary symptoms (urgency, frequency, incontinence, and urinary retention). These drugs are called anticholinergics or antispasmodics and include a number of preparations. The most frequently employed are propantheline bromide (Pro-Banthine and other generic preparations), dicyclomine hydrochloride (Bentyl and other generic preparations), flavoxate hydrochloride (Urispas), hyoscyamine (Cystospaz), and oxybutynin chloride (Ditropan). All of these must be prescribed by a physician, and the dosage monitored for the patient and adjusted if necessary at varying times in the course of the illness. Although there is no conclusive evidence that one anticholinergic agent is superior to another, we have found that patients become less responsive to one after a period of time and then respond to another.

All have the common side effects of this class of drugs: dryness of the mouth, constipation, drowsiness, photophobia (sensitivity to light), and blurred vision. Sometimes it is necessary to accept these side effects in order to achieve the benefits for the bladder. In some cases, complete transient paralysis of the urinary detrusor muscle occurs, which may even be the desired goal to control symptoms. This is discussed later in conjunction with intermittent catheterization.

Some members of another class of drugs, the tricyclic antidepressants, are often useful in the management of uncontrollable urinary muscle contractions. One drug especially, imipramine (Tofranil and other generic preparations), is often used. It has the same side effects as the anticholinergic drugs but is advantageous in that it may be administered once a day because of its long duration of action; it also produces some antidepressant action, which is desirable for some patients.

Another class of drugs—the alpha-adrenergic blocking agents, which

TABLE 3. *Drugs used for bladder control*

Drug	Dose (mg/day)	Tablet size
Pro-Banthine (propantheline bromide)	45–120	15
Ditropan (oxybutynin)	15–45	5
Bentyl (dicyclomine HCl)	30–80	10
Tofranil (imipramine)	25–300	25, 50
Librax (clinidium and chlordiazepoxide)	1 capsule 6–8 times a day	Clinidium, 2.5 mg and chlordiazepoxide (Librium), 5 mg

act on the autonomic nervous system—has also been tried. One drug, phenoxybenzamine (Dibenzyline), is believed by some physicians to be of use in relaxing the bladder muscle in certain cases. It is said to be useful in relaxing the sphincter muscle of the bladder to relieve functional obstruction to urinary outflow. Its major side effect is orthostatic hypotension (it lowers the blood pressure when the patient is standing).

Urecholine is sometimes used for the treatment of urinary retention. It makes the detrusor muscle contract and expel urine. We do not recommend routine use of this agent, as many MS patients have urinary sphincters that do not relax and open properly during urination. Giving urecholine to such a patient would result in the detrusor trying to expel urine against a closed sphincter.

Infections are common and should be treated with specific antibiotics. The infecting organism should be identified, and the specific antibiotic to combat it determined. Sometimes long-term prophylaxis to urinary tract infection is attempted by the use of nitrofurantoin (Macrodantin or Furadantin), nalidixic acid (Negram), sulfonamides (Gantrisin or Gantanol), or a sulfonamide mixed with another drug (Bactrim or Septra). Trimethoprim (Trimpex) may be used in patients who are allergic to sulfa. Drugs for urinary tract infection should be administered only under careful medical supervision.

64 DRUG THERAPY

Other drugs used to prevent urinary tract infection are methenamine hippurate (Hiprex or Urex) and methenamine mandelate (Mandelamine). These may be given for long periods of time at a dose of 2.0 g daily in divided dosage for the methenamine hippurate or 4.0 g in divided dosage for the methenamine mandelate. These drugs are effective as urinary tract antiseptics only in an acidic urine. They are therefore given in conjunction with vitamin C (ascorbic acid), 4.0 g daily in divided dosage (Chapter 11).

Immunosuppressive Therapy

One of the most promising and controversial areas of drug treatments for MS is that of immunosuppression. Since it seems to be apparent that there is an abnormal action of the body's immune system, i.e., lymphocytes, that mediate damage to the nervous system in MS, then it makes sense that an agent that reduces the number and/or type of lymphocytes would slow down or prevent future destruction of myelin. There are currently three immunosuppressive drugs that are commonly used to treat MS patients. These are azathioprine (Imuran), cyclophosphamide (Cytoxan), and cyclosporin (Sandimmune).

Azathioprine has been used for several years in Europe and in this country. Some scientific studies have shown that azathioprine stops progression of MS in patients; other studies have not shown benefit from this agent. Our experience with azathioprine appears to indicate that it stabilizes disease progression in approximately 60% of progressive MS patients in a nonrandomized, noncontrolled trial. The possible side effects of azathioprine include nausea, vomiting, liver toxicity, and long-term increased risk of certain malignancies. The drug also may cause birth defects and should not be given to women who are pregnant or planning to become pregnant.

An agent that more recently has been used in MS patients is cyclophosphamide. One study that compared a group of chronic progressive patients who were treated with cyclophosphamide to a nontreated control group indicated that most of the treated group of patients had stabilization of their disease for up to 1 year. Further controlled trials of this drug are currently in progress. The drug is given intravenously and requires a 3- to 4-week hospitalization. All patients who receive the drug experience total alopecia, which is temporary. The other possible side effects are similar to those of azathioprine (Imuran) and also include bleeding into the bladder, increased risk of infection, and increased risk of future malignancy.

Cyclosporin is an immunosuppressive drug that is being widely used in patients receiving organ transplants. It appears to have a specific suppressant action on the lymphocyte subpopulation that augments the immune response of other lymphocytes. Controlled, double-blind trials of cyclosporin in MS patients are currently in progress. There are no published studies to date showing benefit. Risks include possibility of liver or kidney damage, susceptibility to certain viral infections, and high blood pressure.

In summary, immunosuppressive medications may prove to be an effective means of altering the course and subsequent long-term disability in some patients with MS. To date, however, none of these agents has been proven to have clear benefit, and they have a number of potentially dangerous side effects. Ongoing and future experimental research will indicate if these therapies have a place in the routine treatment of MS patients.

Other Experimental Agents

There are several pharmaceutical agents that are currently being tested in limited trials in this country and abroad. They have not been definitely proven to be of benefit to MS patients and are not yet available to the public. Nonetheless, some preliminary reports seem promising, and so these agents are included.

4-Aminopyridine

4-Aminopyridine has been reported to produce transient (e.g., lasting 30–60 min) improvement in symptoms in some MS patients. This drug is believed to act by facilitating conduction through damaged nerves. Controlled trials are in progress.

Monoclonal Antibodies

Monoclonal antibodies are antibodies to specific classes of lymphocytes. They bind to the lymphocytes and render them inactive. Thus, these antibodies act as immunosuppressive agents. Experiments in mice have shown that monoclonal antibodies prevent the development of an MS-like disease in these animals; patient trials are currently being conducted.

Interferon

Interferon is a substance produced by the body in response to infection by viruses and other agents. An early noncontrolled study in 10 MS patients reported a decrease in number of exacerbations. Further studies are in progress.

Copolymer

This is a synthetic molecule that is immunologically similar to some components of myelin. Early trials indicated a decrease in number of exacerbations in patients with the relapsing–remitting form of the disease. Further double-blind trials in patients with progressive disease are currently ongoing.

Colchicine

Colchicine is an antiinflammatory agent (usually used to treat gout) that has been reported to be effective in preventing the development of an MS-like disease in animals. Pilot studies in humans are being conducted.

7

Treatment with Diet

James Q. Simmons and Barbara S. Giesser

A frequent question posed by those with MS is: Can I eat some special things that will make me well? Is there a diet that will help my MS? The immediate answer of course is that many diets for MS, often claiming cures, have in past years been promoted by doctors and others. Many theories have been advanced to justify diets of various sorts. For example, "The illness is allergic in nature, so eliminate foods to which many are sensitive." "There are deficiencies of minerals, vitamins, or hormones." "There is too much fat in the diet—or perhaps too little; therefore, fatty foods in the diet must be reduced, changed in content, or even, as thought at one time, increased."

Although there have been a variety of different diets proposed for the treatment of MS over the years, each with its own rationale, no properly controlled scientific study has ever unambiguously demonstrated that the course of MS can be influenced by dietary modification. Furthermore, adherence to so-called "curative" dietary regimens may actually do more harm than good, for the following reasons. First, patients may follow a diet that may totally eliminate a vital food group, such as protein, fats, or certain vegetables, and thus deny themselves the nutritional advantages of a balanced diet. Second, "fad" diets may promote practices that are actually harmful, such as megadoses of vitamins. Too much vitamin B_6, for example, can actually cause symptoms that are similiar to those seen in MS, i.e., burning, numbness, and weakness. Finally, a patient may spend valuable time and money on a worthless dietary "cure," thus denying himself proper medical treatment.

This is not to say that there is no place for nutrition in the management of MS. The MS patient functions best when his general health is good. To that end, a balanced, nutritionally sound diet is essential in helping to maintain general good health, promote resistance to infection, aid in wound repair, prevent skin breakdown, and assist in bowel and bladder hygiene.

GENERAL HEALTH

It may appear ludicrous when speaking of someone with MS to emphasize maintenance of a high level of general health. He has MS! But one with MS can be in good health or in poor health. One may fail to lead a healthy, reasonably active life and be in poor general health. He may neglect oral and general hygiene, proper nutrition, elimination, and insistence on living as fully as possible. He may become dependent. As for the diet, it should contain in balanced proportion each of the food groups: meat, vegetable–fruit, milk, and bread–cereal groups.

ESSENTIAL FOOD ELEMENTS

Food elements required for good health are found in these groups: protein, carbohydrates, fats, minerals, vitamins, and water. No single food gives every element or quantity needed. Different groups provide the entire spectrum of needs to work as a team for a good mix of all that is necessary for vigorous health.

To determine the quantity of food needed, we use the unit of food energy produced by foods used in the body, the calorie. One gram of protein or carbohydrate contains 4.5 calories; fat contains a troublesome 9 calories. The food types needed for good body function depend on the level of physical activity. Table 1 shows examples of this difference in food required with differences in activity level. If food is taken in excess of the requirements of these activities, there is fat build-up and obesity. Overweight places a strain on muscles and the heart, and body efficiency suffers.

TABLE 1. *Burning of calories for the average (154-lb) male*

Portion of food	Calories	Activity burns it up if we			
		Recline for	Walk for	Swim for	Run for
Butter, a pat	50	38 min	10 min	4.5 min	2.5 min
Large egg, one	80	61 min	15 min	7 min	4 min
Donut, one	125	1 hr 35 min	24 min	11 min	6 min
Beer, 12 oz	150	1 hr 55 min	29 min	13 min	8 min

From (1965): *J. Am. Diet Assoc.*, 46:186–188.

Protein

Important building blocks for tissue repair are derived from what we eat. There are eight "essential" amino acids; these are not manufactured in the body as other amino acids are. Foods containing the eight "essential" amino acids are meats, fish, and eggs and are considered to be of high nutritional value. Beans, peas, and cereals contain protein of lesser value. Mixtures of the two types, however, make for tasty, less expensive meals.

Some animal food is necessary for a plentiful supply of protein. It is needed for growth, tissue repair, hemoglobin (the protein in the blood that carries oxygen from the lungs to tissues and then carries carbon dioxide from the tissues back to the lungs so it can be eliminated), and for disease-fighting antibodies.

Carbohydrates

Carbohydrates come as starches, sugars, and celluloses and fulfill our greatest energy needs. Cellulose, or plant fiber, has few calories but is necessary for normal bowel action. Adequate fiber or roughage in the diet is important to our lower bowel health.

Glucose, or blood sugar, is digested carbohydrates and, when absorbed into the blood, furnishes energy for body functions and growth. Carbohydrate saves protein for cell repair and helps in the breakdown of fat.

Starchy grains are eaten in pasta, bread, and cereal. Potatoes, sweet potatoes, dry beans, peas, and all the green vegetables also contain carbohydrates. Roughage or stool bulk is derived from wholegrain cereals, vegetables, and fresh or dried fruit.

Fats

Fats are concentrated sources of energy and give twice the energy per gram of protein or carbohydrate. Fats take part in cell structure, cushion vital organs against trauma, and contain essential fatty acids.

Linoleic acid, not produced from other fats in the body, must be provided by our food, and it is found in many oils (corn, cottonseed, safflower, sesame seed, and soybean) and in wheat germ—all polyunsaturated fats. Margarine and cooking oils come from these. Poultry fat and fish oils have more linoleic acid than do other sources.

It is best to keep the total amount of fat ingested moderate and to include sources of polyunsaturated fat. In addition to the oils above, fats are found in cream, cheese, nuts, chocolate, eggs, and meats.

Minerals and Vitamins

The best place to obtain minerals and vitamins is in the food you eat.

Calcium is plentiful in the body. With phosphorus, it gives hardness to teeth and bones, where 99% of the body content of calcium resides. The small amount in other tissues and fluids ensures functioning of the heart, muscle, and nerves and the coagulation of blood. Milk products are an excellent source, as are green vegetables and canned salmon (the kind with bones in).

Iodine prevents goiter and is found in seafood and in today's table salt.

Iron is needed in the formation of hemoglobin. Its content is very high in organ meats (liver, heart, and kidney), shellfish, egg yolk, green vegetables, and dried beans and peas.

Magnesium and *phosphorus* are important for bony structures and are found in whole-grain products and dried peas and beans. If meals contain enough protein and calcium, phosphorus will automatically be contained in the diet. Another 10 minerals needed in trace amounts will also be obtained if foods giving the minerals named above are eaten.

Vitamins play a dynamic role in body functions, in the release of energy from food, in promoting normal growth, and in ensuring proper functioning of all tissues. They are best obtained from foods.

Vitamin A is needed for normal growth and vitality, and it keeps the skin and inner linings of the body healthy. Outstanding sources of A are liver, eggs, whole milk, cheese, and the green and yellow vegetables.

There are many *B vitamins,* and they are called collectively the B-complex vitamins. They are all contained in brewer's yeast. They release energy from food, help the nervous system to function, and are generously supplied in the meats we eat.

Vitamin D builds strong bones and teeth and functions in the body's utilization of calcium and phosphorus. Salmon, sardines, tuna, liver, and egg yolk are the best sources. Vitamin D is also produced in the skin under the influence of the sun and is absorbed in the general circulation.

Vitamin C, or ascorbic acid, maintains the cementing materials that hold body tissues together, strengthens the walls of blood vessels, and assists in the healing processes.

The fact is that no diet for MS to date has been scientifically studied. There are no solid data to study, and we are faced with the unsupported claims of those who have advanced them. Usually claims are advanced with enthusiasm and at times with fanaticism. The claimants all protest, "If I can get the patient on my regimen early enough, my system will work." This statement of course ignores the fact that in the first years of MS there are several disappearances of symptoms, often complete remissions—and occasionally symptoms never return.

Although a specific diet has not been studied, a dietary supplement has been. Seventy-five people with MS were studied in London and Belfast for 2 years using a linoleic acid source for the treated MS patients and an oleic acid source for the "control" MS subjects. Linoleic acid is an unsaturated fatty acid fat; oleic acid is a more saturated one. The investigators reported that the linoleic acid group had fewer acute attacks over the 2-year study, but the progress of the disease was the same in both groups.

Some dietary supplements, such as other unsaturated fatty acid fats, have been added to the diet in a controlled way, and these efforts too have led to disappointment and have failed to show differences in the groups studied.

Perhaps no scientist has come forward with a proposal for diet study in MS because such a study is difficult. It is difficult to plan and carry out. First, the diagnosis of MS in each patient must be confirmed by a special neurological team of doctors to be sure we have a study dealing with MS. For example, in groups referred by community physicians for diagnostic confirmation of MS by neurologists, 35% or more are rejected as not fulfilling the accepted international criteria for an MS diagnosis. Second, it is difficult to keep people on a given diet. Casual eating between meals is an almost unconscious act.

REDUCING DIET

One of the complications faced by MS patients who become increasingly less active is obesity. This extra weight makes it more difficult for them to move or transfer and can predispose to skin breakdown or irritation. Below is an example of a moderate weight reduction diet.

Breakfast

Choose one item from each category:

Fruits and juices
    4 oz juice (preferably cranberry, prune, apricot, or apple)
    1 piece fruit (apple, banana, pear, peach, ½ cup blueberries or strawberries, ½ cup prunes or other stewed fruit, 1 slice melon, 2 or 3 dried figs)

Grains
- 1 slice whole-grain or high-fiber bread
- 1 bran muffin
- 1 English muffin
- ½ hard roll or ½ bagel
- 1 oz high-fiber cereal (bran flakes, all-bran, wheat flakes, shredded wheat, bran and fruit cereals)

Protein
- 1 egg
- 1 oz hard cheese
- 2 oz low-fat cottage cheese
- 1 cup low-fat yogurt (without fruit)
- 1 tablespoon peanut butter

Beverage
- ½ cup low-fat milk
- Coffee or tea

Lunch

Choose one item from each category:

Protein
- 2 oz lean meat (e.g., chicken, beef, turkey, 1 hot dog)
- 2 oz hard cheese
- 2 tablespoons peanut butter
- ⅔ cup low-fat cottage cheese
- 3 oz water-packed tuna or other fish
- 2 eggs

Grains
- 1 slice whole-wheat or high-fiber bread
- 1 pita pocket
- ½ hard roll or bagel
- ½ cup cooked noodles, rice, or pasta
- 10 saltine crackers

Fruits and juices
  Same as for breakfast

Vegetables
  Lettuce, tomato, cucumber, green or red pepper, celery, cabbage, carrots (amounts unlimited, may be eaten in addition to other vegetables)
  ½ cup peas, beans, corn
  1 cup summer squash or ½ cup winter squash

Beverage
  ½ cup low-fat milk
  Coffee, tea, diet soda, bouillon

Dinner

Choose one item from each category:

Protein
  3 oz beef, chicken, fish, lamb, veal, turkey
  2 eggs
  1 cup low-fat cottage cheese
  3 oz hard cheese

Grains
  1 slice whole-wheat or bran bread
  ½ cup cooked rice, pasta, noodles, or buckwheat groats

Vegetables
  ½ cup peas, beans, or mixed vegetables
  1 small ear of corn or ½ cup corn kernels
  1 cup broccoli, cauliflower, squash, eggplant, spinach, or greens
  Lettuce, tomato, pepper, cucumber, celery, carrots, mushrooms (amounts unlimited, these may be eaten in addition to another serving of vegetables)

Dessert or snack
- 1 piece of fruit
- ½ cup gelatin dessert
- 2 cookies (no icing or filling)
- 1 small slice plain cake (no icing or filling)

Beverage
- Coffee, tea, diet soda

This diet supplies approximately 1,200 to 1,300 calories daily. When combined with a program of moderate exercise, it should produce a weight loss that averages 2 lb per week.

General Rules

1. Drink at least 48 to 64 oz of fluid daily, including at least three glasses of water.
2. Do not use additional fats in preparing foods. Trim all fat off of meat, and remove skin from poultry before cooking.
3. You should have at least three servings total of fruits or vegetables daily, including one serving of leafy green vegetable (e.g., lettuce, spinach).
4. Limit eggs to four per week. Try to have at least five fish meals per week.
5. Any weight reduction program is most efficient when combined with a moderate, daily exercise schedule. A beneficial regimen is 20 min of exercise daily, performed within 30 to 60 min of eating a meal. Some experts feel that exercise boosts the body's metabolic rate, enabling it to burn calories more efficiently.
6. Avoid condiments such as mayonnaise, salad dressing, catsup, jams, jellies, and honey. Use mustard, vinegar, lemon juice, and herbs to flavor foods. Artificial sweeteners may be used where appropriate.

SUPPLEMENTAL NUTRITION

For those patients who require additional nutrition, there are several commercially available liquid nutritional supplements that supply protein, calories, and other nutrients. These may be taken in addition to other foods or in place of solid foods. The latter is appropriate for those patients who have difficulty in chewing or swallowing and require feeding tubes.

Patients who are no longer able to chew or swallow food without choking need the placement of a feeding tube. A very small opening in the stomach (gastrostomy) or esophagus (esophagostomy) is made, and a long thin plastic tube is inserted. Any liquid or blenderized diet can be fed through the tubes. They are easy to care for, and patients may be managed at home.

DIET AND URINARY INFECTION

Urinary incontinence may result from urinary tract infection (UTI) or from neurogenic bladder dysfunction, which predisposes the individual to bladder infections. Maintaining an acid urine—a medium unfavorable to the growth of causative organisms—helps prevent UTI. Dietary suggestions to help increase urinary acidity include the following:

1. Protein (meat, fowl, fish, eggs, and gelatin).
2. Large amounts of acidifying cranberries and their juice, plums, and prunes. The cranberry juice provides a vitamin C substitute for citrus juices and is taken throughout the day, since excretion of Vitamin C occurs rapidly. (Intake should be reduced at night to avoid nocturia and nocturnal enuresis.)

The following are foods that MS patients should try to limit in their diet when UTI is a problem: (a) grapefruit, oranges, lemons, tomatoes, and their juices; (b) milk and its products; (c) beverages and antacids containing sodium carbonate or sodium bicarbonate (use Gelusil or other aluminum-type antacids instead); (d) noncitrus fruits

TREATMENT WITH DIET

and vegetables in large quantities, except those listed below; and (e) potatoes, lima beans, soy beans, greens, spinach, and dried vegetables.

As a substitute for potatoes, use two or more servings of white or brown rice, noodles, macaroni, spaghetti, or barley. Use cereals, preferably whole grain, dry, or cooked, and sliced bread, preferably whole grain. For dessert, try prune whips, gelatin, rice custard, bread pudding, tapioca, or custard pie; for nuts, filberts, walnuts, and Brazil nuts. Concentrated sweets may be taken. Fats that may be taken include butter, oil, nut butter, and cooking fats.

ELIMINATION PROBLEMS

Constipation calls for the inclusion of bulk-producing bran combined with the daily use of one of the psyllium seed preparations such as Metamucil; these absorb water and lead to moist stools. Water intake should be adequate. Prunes and prune juice also help reduce constipation.

These dietary measures need to be followed daily, since regulation of the digestive system is involved. If high-fiber intake, prunes, and adequate fluid ingestion do not successfully control constipation after a fair trial period, additional intervention procedures will need to be tried.

CONCLUSION

Adhering to a diet is a discipline, and discipline is a positive force within each of us. If the MS patient accepts this discipline, selects high-nutrient foods, and lives as full and independent and self-sufficient a life as possible, he or she can better deal with the challenges of living and coping with MS.

SUGGESTED READING

The following are available from Superintendent of Documents, U.S. Government Printing Office, Washington, D.C. 20402:

1. *Calories and Weight,* Agriculture Information Bulletin No. 364.
2. *Facts About Nutrition,* DHEW No. (NIH) 74-423-1973, Stock No. 1749-00366.
3. *Food and Your Weight,* Agriculture Information Bulletin No. G 74.
4. *Food for Fitness,* Agriculture Information Bulletin No. L424.
5. *Nutritive Value of Foods,* Agriculture Information Bulletin No. G 72.

8

Physical and Surgical Therapy

Justin Alexander and Ellen Costello

Questions are often asked about the effects of rest, activity, and exercise on multiple sclerosis (MS). Does bed rest help or hinder recovery, especially during an acute attack? What level of activity should be maintained in the weakened or weakening individual? Are there specific benefits to be derived from exercise regimens? To the best of our knowledge, activity or rest has no effect on improving or worsening the disease process itself. However, it may have a definite effect on the more outward changes in the body that come about as a result of the disease. These are sometimes serious complications and can often be prevented by timely use of planned activity and rest. Such a regimen may also help to restore some degree of function and maintain it. The judicious use of various drugs, supportive devices, ambulatory aids, and certain surgical procedures are frequently of added benefit in this context.

There is a general principle that is operative in many individuals with progressive nervous system disorder. It is called "anticipation of disability." This means simply that those who are getting weaker tend to function below their actual capacity. As a matter of fact, it derives from a universal principle. None of us ever work up to our full capacity, a capacity determined by the fact that the human being possesses large untapped reserves of energy. If only half our potential were used normally, and if this tendency continued while our potential were being reduced by disease, we would be left with an insufficient display of energy to maintain an effective level of function. Thus, the MS individual may discontinue extensive activity too early or may even discontinue ambulation too early. The problem is that underusing oneself may lead to the deleterious effects brought on by disuse. The nature of human tissue is such that it reacts to the kind of activity it is called on to perform. If such performance is inhibited, tissue and organs respond by reducing their substance and their function. For example, muscle shrinks (atrophy) and weakens if not used, bone loses its calcium and becomes fragile (osteoporosis), and underinflated lungs become easy prey to infection. This kind of process goes on in all tissues in which normal functioning is reduced or lost. Obviously, if inactivity tends to bring on such problems, activity should be effective in preventing, mitigating, or allaying them.

"Anticipation of disability" may be reinforced by another phenomenon that occurs in MS: the tendency to lassitude and fatigability. Individuals often report that they awaken refreshed in the morning and gradually feel more fatigued as the day passes, reaching a low point sometime in the late afternoon. There often is some recovery of vitality later in the evening. The probable reason for this characteristic cycle is that the fatigue appears to be related to the cycle of change in body temperature during the day. The core temperature of the body is usually lowest in the morning and at night and highest in the late afternoon. Of course, the difference between the lowest and highest points is not very great, and all levels usually are within what is considered the normal range unless the individual has a fever. Minor changes do not matter very much in the normal person, but nerve fibers of the individual with MS that have lost much of their waxy myelin coating in multiple parts of the nervous system are much more sensitive to very small rises in internal temperature. That this is so is shown by the rather remarkable increase in fatigue and the temporary worsening of the condition as determined by examination after being overheated by a hot bath or by the environment on hot, humid days. Because of this phenomenon, individuals who are distressed by feeling fatigued are strongly advised to avoid hot baths and to keep as cool as they can on hot days even though the effects of overheating are only temporary.

Vigorous activity, especially exercising, also raises the internal temperature of the body slightly and may partially account for the rapid fatigue that occurs. For this reason it is advisable to intersperse short bouts of exercise with rest periods of at least equal duration to allow recovery to take place. This principle of exercise–rest–exercise–rest allows for the more effective use of restorative or fitness maintenance programs.

With the foregoing provisos in mind to prevent the abuses of rest, activity, and exercise, we can now discuss their uses. Physical functioning in the person with MS is hindered by weakness, stiffness (spasticity), and loss of coordination (ataxia). Not all necessarily occur at the same time or with the same degree of severity. Therefore, each should be considered separately, even though at times they may tend to reinforce each other in terms of their deleterious effects on function.

WEAKNESS

Loss of strength and endurance is a prominent manifestation of MS. There are various ways in which such a loss can occur. It may be sudden, extensive, and severe (exacerbation), and it may last for days or even weeks, after which the individual may gradually recover (remission). The recovery may not be complete, leaving some residual weakness. Several such episodes may occur, sometimes in rapid succession and sometimes with the lapse of years in between. Alternatively, weakening may be a more gradual and continuing process without remissions. The speed of this process may vary considerably, from extreme rapidity to very slow progression. Fortunately, cases of very rapid progression are rare. On the other hand and more commonly, progression of the disability may be so slow that considerable function is retained for many years.

Cyclical and continuous types occasionally change from one to the other. In fact, there is a wide range of modes of weakening and no sure method of predicting their occurrence. In most instances, the weakness is usually not evenly distributed throughout the body. Both legs may be involved almost equally, or there may be a greater degree of involvement of just one leg. Less frequently, the same is true of the upper extremities. No matter what the type or location of the involvement, in the majority of people the ability to ambulate, even in the weakened state, may be retained for a very long time, especially with continued activity and exercise. The kind of activity and exercise that would be of therapeutic benefit is related to the type and location of the weakening process.

Exercise is most effective when used during recovery from an acute attack, that is, during the remitting stage. The pace and degree of recovery are increased by mobilizing latent potential by means of appropriate exercise. In this sense, the process is restorative. In the slowly and continuously progressive form of MS, exercise is designed to maintain rather than restore strength. In this way, "anticipation of disability" is not allowed to hold sway. In both of these examples, the residual state of the damaged nervous system ultimately dictates the optimal level of function possible as a result of restorative and maintenance programs.

During acute exacerbations and during the rapidly and continuously progressive form of the disease, exercise is much less effective although not harmful. In both cases, the progression of the disability may be more rapid than any benefits to be expected from physical therapy. It must be remembered, however, that total inactivity promotes the appearance of the maximal deleterious metabolic effects of the process of disuse. For example, it is during prolonged periods of bed rest that pressure sores over bony prominences (decubitus ulcers) tend to form because of the poor nutritional status of tissues that normally resist pressure. Unless there is meticulous attention paid to nursing care of the bedridden patient, including frequent turning of the individual with close inspection of the skin over pressure areas, these ulcers are a danger.

If any large group of people with MS were asked the function they would prefer to maintain, the majority would probably choose the ability to walk effectively. There are a number of disorders that place effective walking in jeopardy (such as weakness, spasticity, and loss of coordination). Activities, especially walking, depend on strength, endurance, speed, and coordination.

In order to increase strength, the muscle groups that perform movements must be worked against the heaviest loads they can carry. This must be done against gravity and through the full range of movements. Special attention must be paid to the antigravity muscles, such as those of the calves, front of the thighs, the rear muscles, which straighten the hips, and the muscles of the lower back. It is the weakening of these muscles that makes walking in the erect position so difficult. Because the resistance afforded by externally applied loads is maximal, only a very few repetitions through the complete range of motion can be tolerated. However, even these few repetitions, repeated daily, may be sufficient, providing the damage to the nervous system is not enough to deny improvement of strength. Heavy resistance exercise is quite a popular form of physical therapy and is sometimes done with fans blowing air over exercising MS patients to keep them cool. It must be remembered that the maximal load tolerated depends on the degree of residual strength, being greater in the stronger person and less in the weaker.

Training for endurance must be done differently. Endurance cannot be built up with only a few repetitions of the movements, as training for strength alone does not necessarily provide endurance. Many repetitions are required during exercise to fulfill the need for prolonged activity not requiring great strength, which is the usual situation in daily living. Therefore, the load during these exercises is only a fraction of that required when building up strength. The smaller the load, the more repetitions are possible. Ideally, loads should be chosen that compare to those encountered in the activities of daily living.

It should be obvious from the foregoing that some professional help is needed when the patient is learning how to exercise for building strength and endurance. Therefore, the physician will usually prescribe a few sessions with a skilled physical therapist, who will teach patients how to do these exercises by themselves and in their own homes. They are, of course, designed for individuals who are still strong enough to walk, even though poorly. Such vigorous exercises are often beyond the capacity of the individual who is too weak to walk. The exercises can only improve preexisting movements, not create them.

SPASTICITY

Damage to the central nervous system usually causes some degree of spasticity. Spasticity is caused by involuntary muscle contractions, and the relaxation from these contractions is also involuntary. Spasticity is stimulated by changes in posture, mainly by stretching some muscles and contracting others. This is exactly what happens when the MS patient is walking: the weakened muscles still under voluntary control tend to act in an orderly pattern, some contracting while others relax. While doing so they coincidentally stimulate a pattern of involuntary (spastic) contractions, not an orderly process. Muscles contract excessively here, including those that are supposed to be relaxing. As a result, the individual's gait becomes labored, stiff, and slow because voluntary movement is now fighting involuntary movement.

The added muscle action of spasticity may enable an individual to stand even though voluntary control may be not quite enough to do so by itself. However, because more muscle mass is being used than is necessary for graceful walking, the energy costs are so increased that endurance is markedly reduced. The individual who has sufficient voluntary control, and who would be able to walk more easily, farther, and better without spasticity, will reach an early point of exhaustion with it. In addition, spasticity tends to stiffen knees and hips and push down the feet. The ability to step high enough to clear the feet from the walking surface is lost. This becomes an especially difficult problem when mounting stairs and going uphill. It is also not compatible with skilled use of the arms and hands when, less frequently, the upper extremities become involved in the spasticity process.

Spasticity has become increasingly manageable in recent years thanks to the introduction of reasonably effective antispasticity drugs. Although these agents may not eliminate all stiffness, by titrating the dosage they may reduce spasticity enough that the individual can function more effectively using less energy. There are a number of drugs that can produce this result, but some have other, less desirable effects as well. They may weaken voluntary motion or excessively tranquilize the individual when given in doses that reduce the spasticity.

Fortunately, there are drugs that concentrate mostly on the spasticity.

Such drugs are begun by the physician in very small doses and then are increased every 3 or 4 days until the best possible effect is obtained. The top dose varies from one individual to another and depends on the severity of the spasticity. When the underlying weakness and the spasticity are both severe, there is a point, when adjusting the dosage, that the legs may become rubbery because support of the spasticity is diminished. The patient's ability to stand and even his labored walking are now jeopardized. This is a signal to revert to the next lower dose. Even the minimal effect of a small dose is valuable, as the individual will quickly discover if the antispasticity drug is completely withdrawn.

A destabilizing effect of the drugs in the individual who is not ambulatory, who has good upper extremities, but who also has very severe and uncomfortable spasticity in the legs is not a major concern. Therefore, large doses can be used in this patient so that he is more comfortable sitting in a wheelchair or lying in bed. The individual with strong underlying voluntary motion, whose gait is awkward and exhausting because of excessive spasticity, should also be given larger doses, as they would not threaten his ability to walk.

With appropriate use of antispasticity medication, walking may be improved still further by supporting the dropped feet. Laminated polyethylene short leg braces are usually prescribed for this purpose. They fit within the shoes and are not unsightly. They keep the toes clear of the ground, further reducing the energy needed to walk.

When weakness and spasticity become excessive, the ability to function is markedly reduced, and the individual tends to be relegated to the wheelchair or may even begin spending much of the day in bed. This creates a vicious cycle because the effects of disuse created by these circumstances reduce function still further. Activity can be maintained in this situation by using underwater activity as therapy. The buoyancy of lukewarm water in a swimming pool eliminates much of the disabling forces of gravity and allows for a degree of function no longer possible on dry land (such as walking). Water also provides some resistance to movement, which is beneficial in enhancing strength. Regular sessions in the swimming pool should be part of the regimen to maintain fitness.

Spasticity, especially when unevenly distributed, may tend to produce deformities that can develop as further barriers to effective walking. In the most common example, the inner thigh muscles sometimes become so excessively hyperactive that gait will take on a scissoring appearance. If the hyperactivity is greater on one side, that leg will be pulled inward, pushing up the pelvis on that side in an attempt to keep the leg in a straight up-and-down posture. This tilting of the pelvis will also curve the spine away from the midline and perhaps throw it off balance. Because of the tilt up, the leg seems to be shorter. When such deformities are sustained over a long time, the muscles gradually adapt their lengths to the distorted postures, and the deformities become more difficult to correct. This deforming propensity of spasticity may occur in other areas as well.

The tendency to deformation must be combated by applying counterbalancing forces regularly. Such forces are supplied by what is known as "passive stretching" exercises. Joints are carried through their full range of motion periodically, making sure that muscles are stretched to their full lengths. This will mitigate against deforming postures being long sustained and prevent them from becoming fixed. The exercises should be done on a daily basis and often require the help of a family member. They are easier to perform when antispasticity drugs are used to lessen the resistance of muscles to stretching.

Occasionally a spastic contraction is so strong that the response to these exercises is less than hoped for. When that occurs, "nerve blocks" may be tried. Injecting an anesthetic around the nerve that leads to the hip weakens those muscles sufficiently that immediately after the block the individual may be able to walk without scissoring and even use less energy. If this proves to be effective in a particular individual, a longer-lasting nerve block with a solution of phenol can maintain the weakening effect for 6 months or longer; it sometimes even has a permanent effect. If the anesthetic does not provide relief, its effect will pass off quickly with no harm done, and another form of management will have to be considered.

Although the inner thigh muscles are useful in walking, they are not absolutely essential. People have been known to walk well with these muscles completely paralyzed. Other excessively contracting muscle groups that can produce deformity may be more important for walking. Fortunately, the technique of temporary nerve blocking can determine very quickly whether walking is possible, and it is a rather simple and not a frightening procedure.

When the deformity is fixed and not reversible through blocking, more radical procedures are called for, such as cutting the tendons of offending muscles. The tendons will rejoin over time but will be of greater length, making the muscles attached to them that much shorter and therefore weaker. This, in a sense, produces a result similar to that of nerve blocking in patients without fixed deformity. The main drawback to cutting tendons is that an overcorrected position must be maintained for several weeks by splints or a plaster cast so that the gap between the cut ends of the tendon will be filled in by the longest possible new tendon. An intensive course of physical therapy immediately following removal of the splints or cast should rapidly reverse the effects of the weeks of inactivity, and the patient should rapidly gain and retain a new and improved pattern of gait.

LOSS OF COORDINATION

Loss of coordination could be a most difficult problem for the person with MS. Fortunately, it does not always occur. When it does, it often does not progress to the point of overwhelming disability, and sometimes it undergoes spontaneous remission. There are no truly effective drugs to control it, and exercise therapy is usually of minimal benefit except perhaps if the loss is mild. Loss of coordination manifests in several ways. Every individual with MS should be familiar with the finger-to-nose and heel-to-shin tests that are performed during the physical examination. The more the arm or leg wavers in performing these tests (intention tremor), the greater the loss of coordination of the upper or lower extremities. When the wavering is only slight, the legs and arms still have their usefulness. This symptom is not always evenly distributed. It can be mild or almost nonexistent in the extremities yet become evident on walking. In that case, the gait would be unstable, with a tendency to stagger to one side or the other, especially on turning; this occasionally leads to a fall.

Above all, gait must be kept within safe limits, and for this purpose walking aids should be used to stabilize locomotion. These aids afford different degrees of stability depending on how broad a supporting base is being offered. If only slight stabilization is needed, a simple cane is enough, usually used on the side toward which the individual staggers. A cane with four supporting points at the base (quad cane) broadens the supporting surface still further and is indicated when greater stabilization is needed. The proper height of a cane is determined by standing upright with the cane held at the side. The height is correct when the elbow is at a 30 degree angle in this position.

Finally, the broadest base affording the greatest degree of stability is provided by a walker. This is a light aluminum structure with two supporting points on either side. Its proper height is determined as it is for a cane. The walker is lifted and advanced prior to each step. The type that can be folded, making it easy to transport, is preferable.

We recently saw a patient who had not walked for 9 years because of an unstable gait. Examination revealed adequate strength and only minimal spasticity and loss of coordination of the arms and legs. There was no evidence that the disease had worsened over these years. Unfortunately, no one had thought of providing her with walking aids. Upon being presented with a walker, she was able to walk safely and for considerable distances with minimal training. This is a glaring example of lost opportunity because of neglect in using walking aids. Fortunately it does not occur often.

There are some who resist the use of aids because they do not like the appearance. They pay the price of staying home with restricted movement because of lack of safety or because they might appear to be intoxicated to others in public. There is no shame in helping oneself, especially if one profits by it with increased activity and widened horizons.

A trial of therapeutic exercise should be considered in all forms of disability including loss of coordination. However, it should not be continued endlessly if there are no favorable results—and such results should become apparent within a few weeks. If gains do occur, however, they cannot be expected to continue forever because that is saying that exercise can restore normality, and, in most cases, that is not possible. When gains are achieved, they should be maintained by self-activation. The best exercise is to use oneself maximally and thus prevent "anticipation of disability." The type of exercise that can be used by the individual with mild to moderate loss of coordination is described later.

NONAMBULANT INDIVIDUAL

To this point we have considered the individual who is still walking to some extent. However, the progression of the disease may reach a point when walking is no longer possible despite every effort to restore and maintain it. Prior to this time and when ambulation has become extremely taxing, the use of a wheelchair for longer distance is called for. This makes the transition to total nonambulation easier and maintains the range of the individual's activities. For those with useful arm motion, wheelchairs can maintain fitness because of the energy demanded to move the chair. If that becomes too exhausting, or if the upper extremities are too weak or uncoordinated to move the chair effectively, various types of battery-powered chairs and vehicles are available. Selection of an appropriate wheelchair requires an evaluation of the person's ability to move, to transfer, the environment in which the person will be using the chair, and a knowledge of what is available. A physical therapist can provide assistance in picking the best chair for any person.

When walking is no longer possible, the ability to propel a wheelchair is not enough. The person must be able to transfer from bed to wheelchair, from wheelchair to another seat (as in theaters, autos, or toilets), and into a shower or bath. To accomplish this, transfer training may be required. The principles underlying such training are simple. They consist of (a) strengthening the muscles of the arms and shoulders so that they can lift the trunk and carry it for short distances, (b) learning what supporting surfaces can be used most effectively in making transfers, (c) learning how to use sliding boards when arms are weak, and (d) moving in the shortest and most direct way, which can be accomplished by placing the wheelchair at an angle to the bed or chair. Often transfer maneuvers can be done by the patient himself, although occasionally some assistance is required. If the patient has maintained a range of locomotion and the ability to transfer himself, work and avocational and recreational pursuits should be restricted only minimally.

OTHER EXERCISE REGIMENS

No discussion of the uses of exercise would be complete without mentioning certain special types that have their enthusiastic advocates. Chief among them are facilitation and biofeedback exercises. Facilitation exercises comprise a number of systems most often labeled with the names of the originators of the systems. They are quite complex and require experienced therapists for their application.

Despite their apparent variety, a common principle governs all of them. When the central nervous system has been damaged, it tends to become overly excitable. That is the basis for the development of spasticity. The hyperexcitable nervous system responds to many kinds of stimulation, which in normal circumstances it would not do. The response consists largely of muscle contraction.

The facilitation exercise systems are based on the fact that certain muscles that enhance desired movements respond to the right kind of stimuli at the right places. Stimuli are supplied by changes in the posture of specific parts of the body or by brushing or tapping certain skin areas. There is a doctrine developed around the relationship among the kinds of stimuli, the place to be stimulated, and the specific muscles that will respond.

Unfortunately, there is no clear-cut evidence that increased strength, endurance, and range of voluntary movement result from the facilitation exercises. Nevertheless, practitioners of these methods often claim good results. For this reason, they may be worth a therapeutic trial during a stable period (remission). Proponents of this technique suggest that "plasticity" of the nervous system permits motion elicited through enforcement to eventually become voluntary and thereby functional.

Biofeedback training is of more recent vintage. It is based on the amplification of electrical signals produced by muscle contraction so that the individual can see the result of even minimal voluntary contraction on a television-like screen or hear the signals from a loudspeaker. Seeing and hearing small contractions, even those that are insufficient to produce any meaningful movement, is a motivating force in attempting to increase the size and volume of what is being seen and heard, and so perhaps to achieve increased movement. It is really a refinement of exercise therapy where more visible small movements motivate the individual to strive for larger ones. It is also used in an attempt to inhibit excessive muscle activity as in spasticity. Unfortunately, its role in treatment is not yet clearly established. After all, it is meant to enhance existing voluntary motion, not to create it. It does not have the magical ability to translate involuntary to voluntary motion. Ultimately, the remaining intact part of the nervous system will determine what is possible, and that can be done in most cases by more traditional forms of physical therapy.

In summary, there is a role for exercise therapy in restoring or maintaining function. The extent to which this is possible is limited by the nature and degree of damage to the nervous system, by the severity of weakness, spasticity, and incoordination, and by fatigability. The tendency to anticipate disability that leads to the constitutional effects of disuse is reversible. Exercise therapy is designed to increase strength, endurance, speed, and coordination. The use of certain drugs, nerve blocks, supporting devices, walking aids, and occasionally surgery may be of help in this process. The major role of self-help and self-activation is emphasized. To this end, a personal exercise regimen is outlined.

PERSONAL EXERCISE REGIMEN

Length of muscles can be maintained by ensuring that all joints of limbs are moved through their complete range at least once daily. It may, however, require more than one attempt to gain this objective. The exercises can be done independently or, if necessary, with the aid of other persons. The exercises described here are only examples of a whole host of activities that can be used to achieve the treatment objectives. A practical program should consist of no more than 10 to 15 exercises, each repeated 10 to 20 times per session, and should not last more than 20 minutes per session. If possible, exercises may be performed several times during the day, preferably at the same time so that exercising becomes a regular daily routine. The program should be carefully designed to meet the needs of the individual based on an evaluation of the patient's muscle strength and range of motion. Different starting positions may be used to permit muscles to function at their optimal efficiency, having gravity act as a resistive force, as assistance, or by neutralizing the effect completely. A firm surface, such as the floor or mat table, will make exercising more effective.

Exercising in a pool can also be beneficial, since buoyancy of the water can be used to initiate motion where muscle power may be inadequate to perform exercises under other conditions. The temperature of the water can serve to reduce spasticity or to increase tone. It is important to note that heat has a tendency to cause fatigue, and excessive fatigue can be harmful.

Generally, exercises should be done on one side and repeated on the other unless they are designated as symmetrical or bilateral or if muscle strength of one side differs markedly from the other. Exercises should always be done slowly and should extend through the entire range of motion. Routines should be modified to accommodate for change in the patient's general condition and should also be altered from time to time to avoid boredom. A physical therapist can design a program to fit the needs of the patient and can incorporate the desired effects into recreational and/or other purposeful activities. Periodic physical therapy evaluation and updating of the home treatment program is as important as the regular follow-up by the physician.

Facelying, Preferably on a Firm Surface

1. Bend the knee to 90° and lift the leg 3 to 5 inches off the supporting surface, hold to the count of five, and return to the starting position (Fig. 1). Twisting or rotating the trunk should be avoided.

If help is required, the assistant should cradle the leg in one arm and press with the other hand on the patient's buttock to ensure that the motion occurs at the hip joint. If the goal of exercising is to strengthen the muscles, resistance should be applied. This can take the form of pressure exerted by the "helper" on the buttock (for stabilization) and over the back of the knee joint. Resistance should

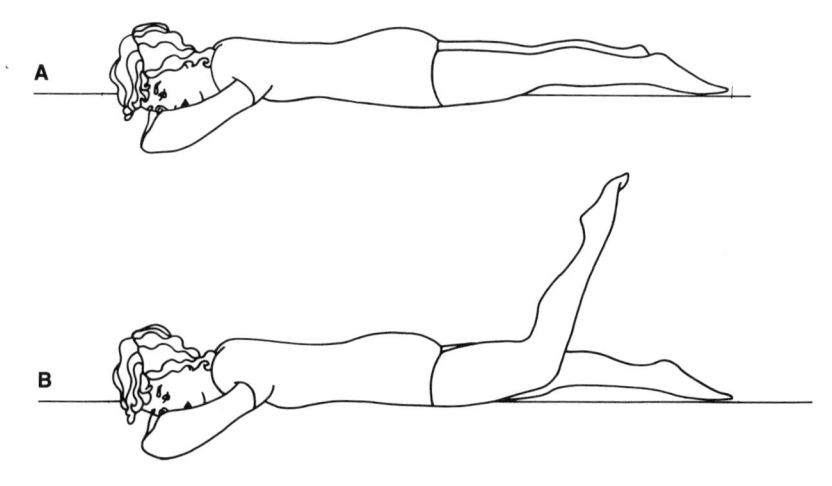

FIG. 1.

not be so heavy as to prevent motion but enough to constitute a challenge.

Resistance can also be applied by means of a sand bag, a bag filled with canned goods, or other easily available objects. An exercise boot with plate weights can be obtained from any store that sells sporting goods. "Cuff weights" are very easy to use for almost any body part. Some have provisions for varying the weight.

2. Keeping the hip and buttocks fixed, bend the knee back. Normal range is about 110° to 120° from the fully straightened position. If assistance is required, stabilization should be provided over the hip and back of the thigh, cradling the lower leg. This ensures better control of motion. Manual resistance can be applied over the back of the ankle, and a pulley with weights can also be employed to provide resistance.

3. Holding on to a fixed point with the arms extended over the head, attempt to lift both legs 3 to 5 inches off the supporting surface. This is an excellent exercise to strengthen low back muscles. This exercise should not be attempted if the back muscles are stiff or tight.

4. With arms resting along the body, lift both arms about 10 inches off the surface (Fig. 2). Some find it helpful to hold on to a stick.

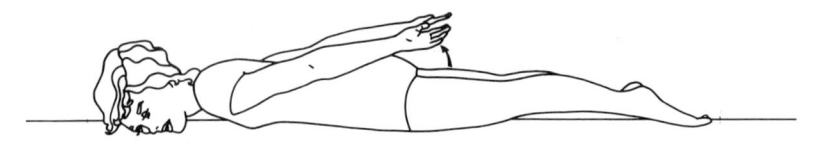

FIG. 2.

This is especially recommended when one arm is weaker. If assistance is required, one arm at a time is exercised. Stabilization should be applied over the shoulder, and the arm should be cradled. Manual resistance can be applied over the elbow, and of course the patient can hold any type of weight in the hand.

5. With hands clasped behind the low back, squeeze shoulders together and attempt to lift the head and shoulders from the surface (Fig. 3). Exercise can be made more challenging by clasping the hands behind the head and finally by holding a weight in that fashion.

6. Push-ups: place both hands on the floor at the level of the shoulder and slowly straighten both elbows, thereby raising head, chest, and as much of the trunk as possible from the floor. Hold to a count of five and slowly lower the body back to the floor.

A modified push-up requires only the raising of head and upper trunk.

Hands and Knees Position

1. Lower the head and simultaneously round the back by tightening stomach muscles (Fig. 4A,B). Then raise the head and allow the back to sag down, giving a swayback appearance (Fig. 4C).

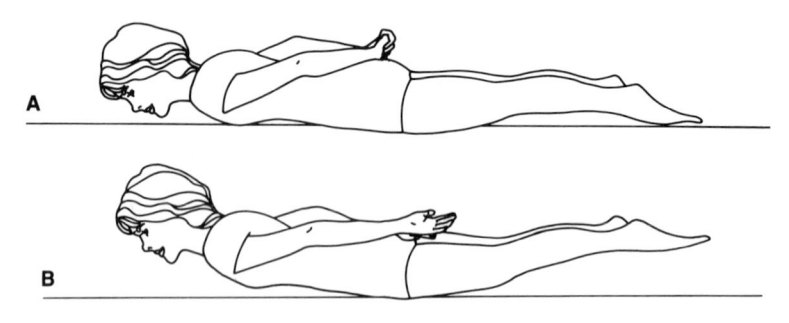

FIG. 3.

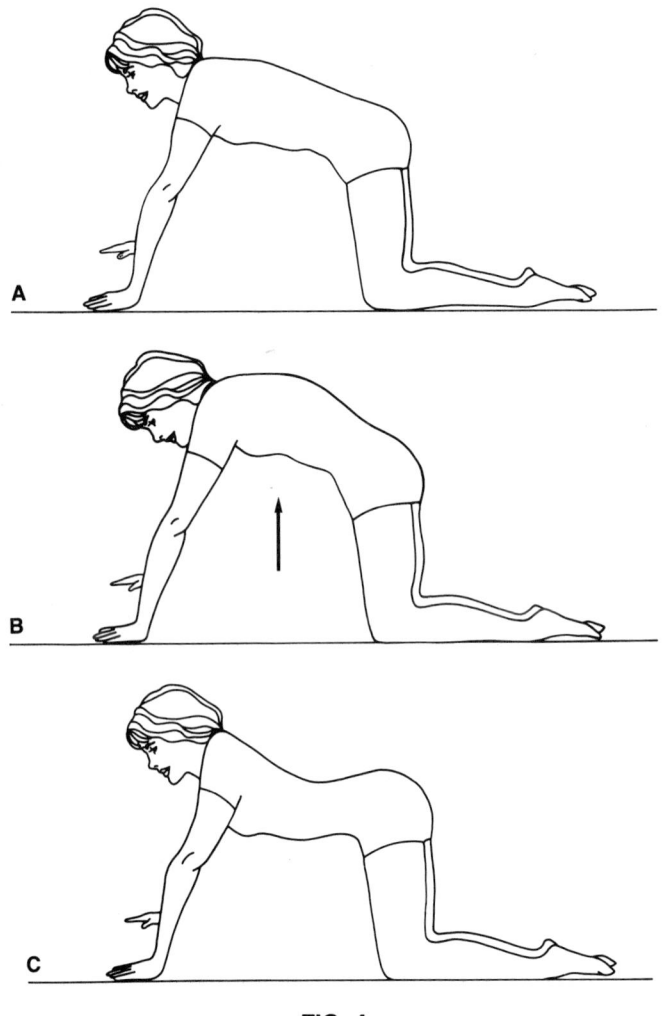

FIG. 4.

2. Balance exercise. (a) Head up: shift weight to right; divide weight bearing on all fours; shift weight to the left. (b) Head up: shift weight to right and raise left arm; lower arm; shift weight to all fours; shift weight to left; raise right arm. (c) Head up: lift left arm and right leg; relax; lift right arm and left leg. (d) Raise trunk to kneeling position; lift arms to side or forward. Assistant may gently push against the trunk to increase balance response.

Backlying

1. Straight leg raising: with arms at the side, lift each leg as high as possible and pull toes and foot towards the trunk (Fig. 5). Both knees should be kept straight, and the small of the back should stay flat against the floor.

If assistance is required, stabilization occurs over the pelvis, and the leg should be cradled. If the posterior thigh muscles (hamstrings) are tight and need to be stretched, the assistant should kneel in front of the patient, place the patient's leg on his (the assistant's) shoulder, clasp his hands over the patient's knee, and slowly straighten up while maintaining pressure over the knee.

This same exercise can be modified to increase the strength of the hip flexors by stabilizing over the pelvis and offering manual resistance over the knee. Weights can be used quite easily for this purpose.

2. Spread the legs apart, symmetrically when possible. A variation of this exercise involves hooking one leg over the edge of the bed or any other fixed point and moving the other leg.

If assistance is required, the helper can move one leg at a time,

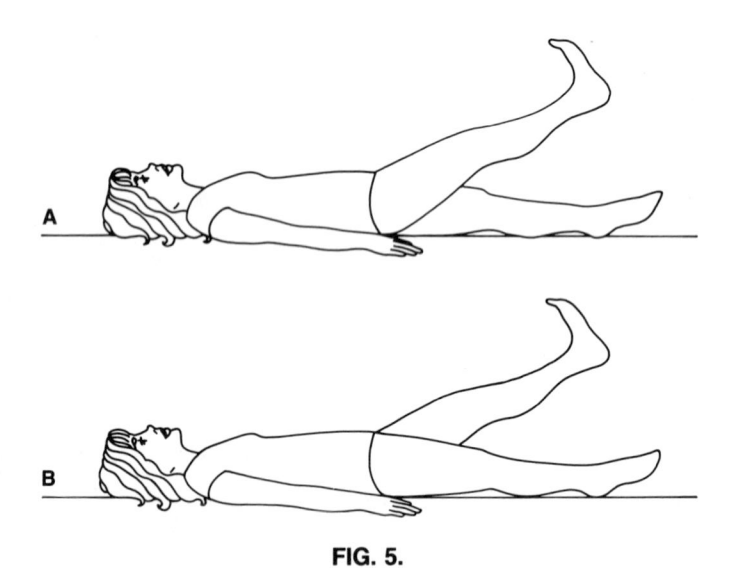

FIG. 5.

cradling the moving leg and holding the other one; or he can grasp both heels and then move the legs apart. Some people find it easier to kneel between the patient's legs and push with their own legs to stretch the adductors.

Spreading the legs can be used for several purposes. If inner thigh muscles (adductors) are tight, stretching can be achieved in this manner. Resistance to spreading the legs can be used to increase muscle strength necessary to maintain a level pelvis, thus enabling standing, or to move the leg out to the side (abductors). When both legs are moved simultaneously, resistance is given on the outer aspect of the ankle. If one leg is moved at a time, stabilization of the pelvis with one hand is essential. Resistance can be applied at the outer aspect of the knee.

3. Sit-ups can be used to strengthen abdominal muscles. Knees should be bent and held firmly by the assistant. If no assistant is available, the feet can be hooked under a firm support (low couch). Exercise should initially be performed with the arms straight out in front, lifting the head and shoulders up (Fig. 6). It is important that the head be kept well forward at all times. The exercise can be progressed by folding the arms over the chest and finally behind the back of the head.

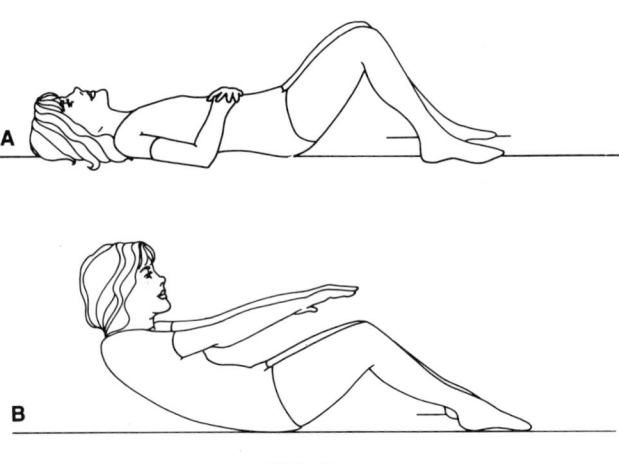

FIG. 6.

98   PHYSICAL AND SURGICAL THERAPY

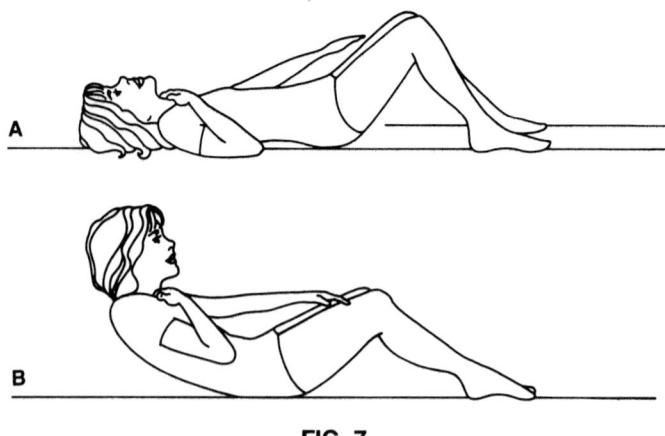

FIG. 7.

4. Place the right hand on the left shoulder, extending the left arm (Fig. 7A). As the body is raised, the left arm reaches toward the right hip and knee (Fig. 7B). Repeat to the opposite side: with left hand on right shoulder and right arm extended, sit up and reach toward left hip and knee. This is a modification of the sit-up that can be performed to include trunk rotator muscles.

5. Bend both knees, plant feet firmly against the floor, and raise buttocks off the floor (Fig. 8).

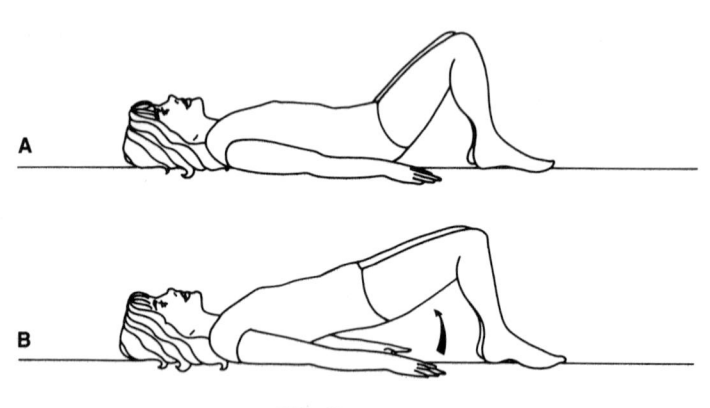

FIG. 8.

FIG. 9.

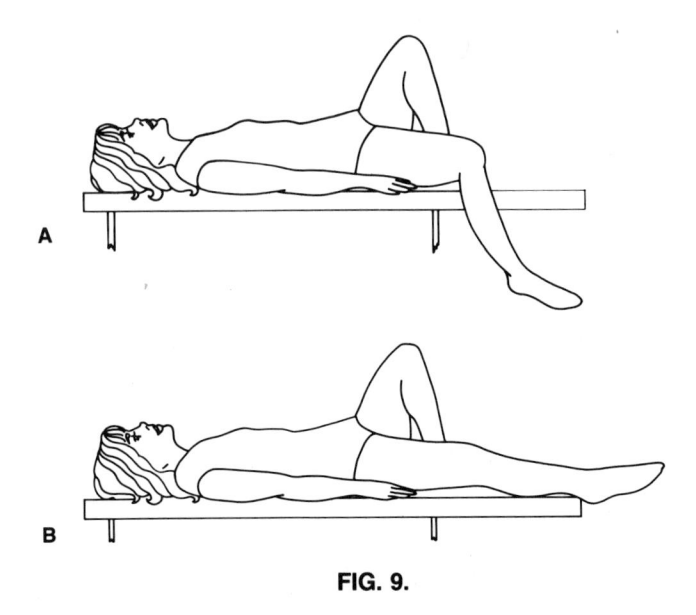

6. Move to the edge of a raised surface until one leg can be bent at the knee over the edge of the table; the other leg is then raised until the foot can rest on the surface (Fig. 9A). Straighten the leg hanging over the edge of the table (Fig. 9B).

Resistance can be applied by a weighted boot, cuff weight, pulleys with weight, or an assistant. In the latter case, the helper pushes against the leg just in front of the ankle. When using mechanical resistance, a small towel roll under the knee being exercised is quite helpful. If muscle goes into spasm, do not attempt this exercise.

7. Bend toes and ankle toward the head as if standing on the heel (Fig. 10). This stretches the heel cord and can be used to increase the strength of the muscles that allow ambulation without stubbing one's big toes (dorsiflexors). Resistance can be supplied by the assistant's hand over the top of the foot, by sand bags, or by cuff weights.

8. Hold onto a stick with both hands, and let arms lie straight along the body. Raise both arms as high as possible above the head, keeping the elbows straight. An assistant can help to continue the motion if muscle tightness prevents reaching the target. To use this

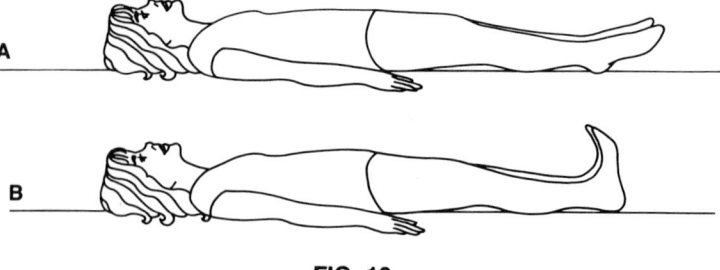

FIG. 10.

exercise for strengthening, plate weights, sand bags, or cuff weights can be attached to the stick.

9. Hold on to a stick and, with elbows bent and hands next to the shoulders, push up to the ceiling. Resistance can be added as described above.

Sitting in a Wheelchair

One of the most important exercises to be performed by the person confined to a wheelchair is designed to provide relief for the buttocks and thus avoid pressure sores. An additional benefit is strengthening the triceps muscles.

1. Place hands on the armrests of the chair and straighten the elbows (Fig. 11). Hold to the count of three and slowly lower the body back into the seat. The whole body can be raised from the chair in this fashion. Guard against allowing the shoulders to be elevated. If the legs cannot be raised concomitantly with the rest of the body, just raising the buttocks off the seat will do, as will shifting pressure from buttock to buttock by leaning side to side. This exercise should be performed at least five to 10 times every hour while sitting up.

2. Arms in lap; raise arms as high as possible and breathe in deeply. Let arms down and exhale.

3. With the arms straight toward the floor, bend the arm, bringing the hand toward the shoulder. Resistance can be offered by means of various weights and pulleys or by an assistant who places one hand just proximal to the elbow, holding the upper arm steady and giving resistance over the wrist.

PHYSICAL AND SURGICAL THERAPY

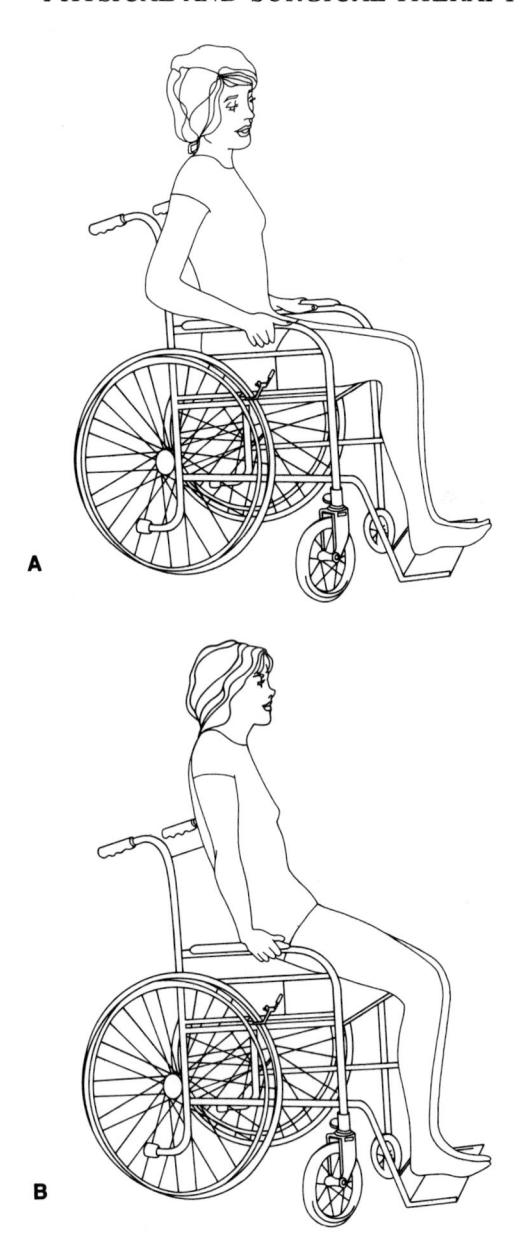

A

B

FIG. 11.

4. Raise one knee at a time toward the chest. Keep the trunk steady. Hold to a count of three and let the leg down. Repeat with other leg. Resistance can be given by means of a weighted boot, sand bag, or cuff weights. An assistant can apply pressure over the thigh just above the knee.

5. Straighten the knee until the lower leg and thigh are in a straight line. If muscle tightness interferes with this motion, rest one leg on a chair (with a cushion under the heel to prevent skin breakdown) and place a weight over the knee. Allow the muscle to stretch for about 15 to 20 minutes. It is important to sit straight.

If resistance is needed, a weighted boot, sand bag, or cuff weights can be used. An assistant places one arm under the exercising knee, resting a hand on the stationary knee, and provides resistance by pushing against the lower leg just above the ankle.

6. Place the heel of one leg over the ankle of the other. Slide heel to the knee and down. Watch the leg closely while performing the exercise. Try the same exercise with eyes closed.

Modify the above exercise by raising the heel from the other leg and placing it at preselected points of the leg. The assistant can touch the point to which the heel is to be raised. First use visual guidance, and then attempt it without watching.

7. Throw and catch a ball, either a beach ball, basketball, or medicine ball, depending on the strength of the patient. Variations of the exercise may include: (a) Hold the ball in both hands with elbows at shoulder level, push the ball away. (b) Hold the ball in both hands, raise arms above head, throw the ball. (c) Hold the ball in one hand at the side of the chair, throw the ball; the other hand may be used to maintain balance by holding on to the chair.

Standing

1. While holding on to a stable support (avoid coffee tables, etc.), stand on one leg, if possible with knee slightly bent, and raise yourself on your toes (Fig. 12). Repeat until the exercise can be performed 10 times. If this causes muscle spasm, avoid the exercise.

2. Place a series of adhesive tape strips on the floor about 12 to 18 inches apart in a staggered fashion to provide a guide for placing the feet when walking. Attempt to walk, touching each piece of tape with the leading foot.

3. Dance to slow music. This is an excellent way of improving balance.

Selection of specific exercises should be based on the particular need of an individual. It is best to select a limited number of the most important exercises to be done at one time. Exercising must be built into the daily schedule as much as any other normal activity. The program should be reviewed periodically by the physical therapist to ensure that it is still correct and to permit modifications.

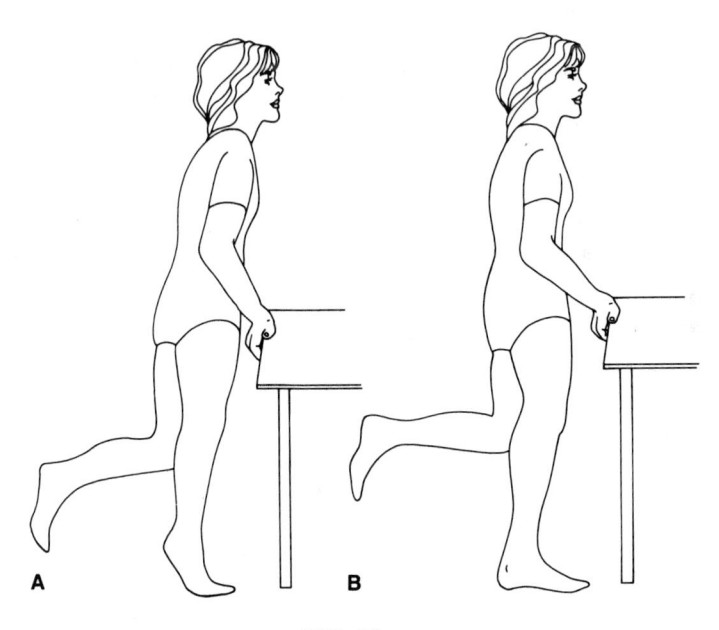

FIG. 12.

STRETCHING EXERCISES

Stretching may be used to minimize or overcome muscle tightness and joint limitation and to decrease spasticity. When stretching, it is important that all motion, whether active (by the patient) or passive (by a helper), be performed slowly and into the "tightness." The muscle should be held in the stretched position to the count of three and then released slowly. Many of the exercises described may be used for stretching. A few examples of special "stretching exercises" are given.

Backlying

1. With the patient lying on a firm surface, the assistant straddles one leg, lifting the other on his/her shoulders, clasping the hands over the patient's elevated knee and then gradually raising the patient's leg by assuming a more upright position (Fig. 13). Hold; when resistance decreases, take up the slack; then release.

2. With the patient lying on a firm surface, both hips are flexed to the maximum by hugging the knees to the chest (Fig. 14A). Alternately, one leg is extended while the opposite leg is held firmly (Fig. 14B). An assistant may provide stabilization by holding the knee onto the

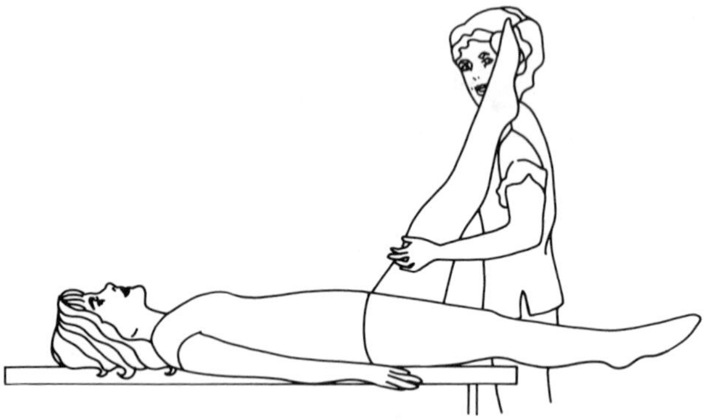

FIG. 13.

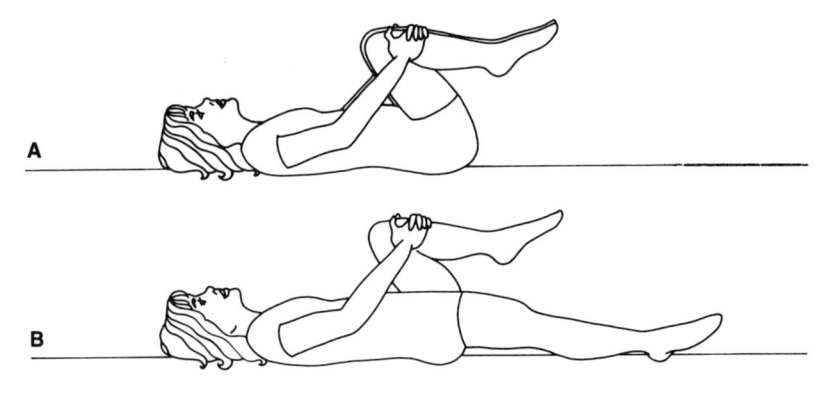

FIG. 14.

chest and increase the stretch by gently pushing on the extended leg.

3. With the patient lying on a firm surface, both knees are bent and then slowly pushed to the side (Fig. 15), stretching the inside of the thigh (adductors).

4. Assistant firmly grasps the heel of the foot, resting the bottom of the foot against his/her forearm, and slowly and firmly pulls on the heel cord, bending the entire foot towards the trunk (Fig. 16).

5. Standing, keep one leg slightly flexed and place both hands against a wall. Bend arms, allowing body to move towards wall while keeping heel firmly on the floor (Fig. 17). A variation of this exercise involves keeping both legs straight.

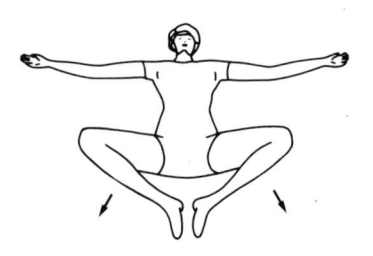

FIG. 15.

106   PHYSICAL AND SURGICAL THERAPY

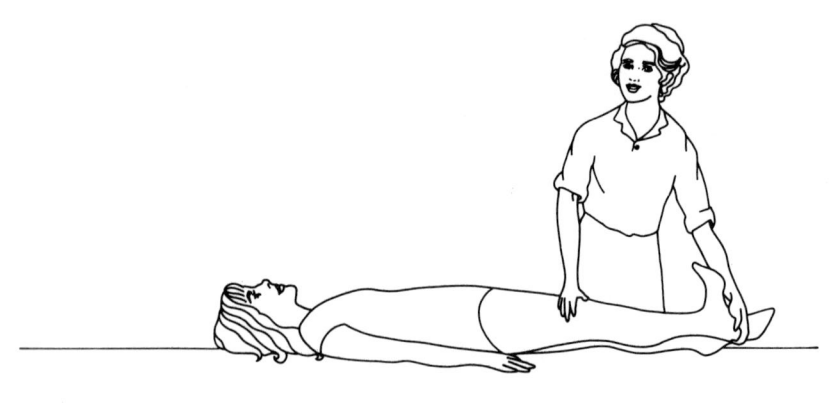

FIG. 16.

6. Sitting, fold hands behind the head and push elbows towards the back. If necessary, an assistant can increase the stretch by standing behind the patient and gently pulling backwards at the elbows.

7. With elbows at shoulder level, press palms together; follow with same exercise but pressing the backs of the hands together (Fig. 18).

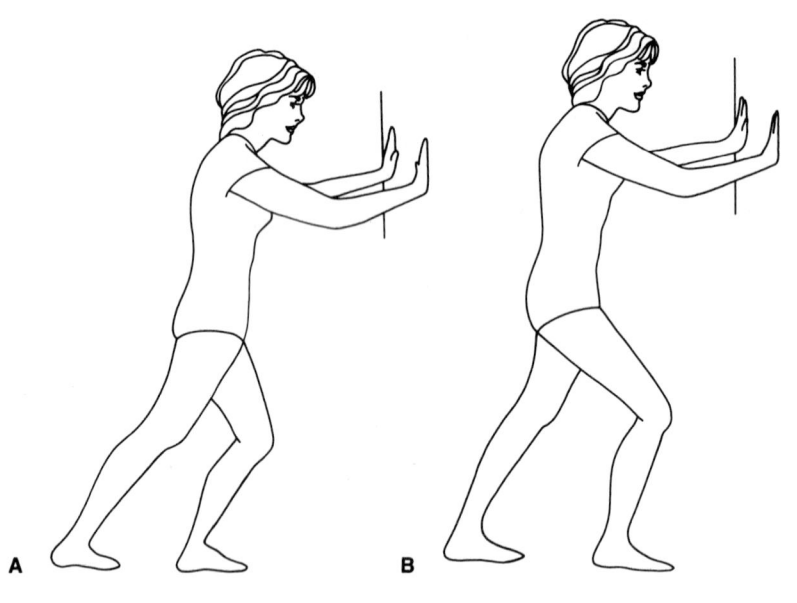

FIG. 17.

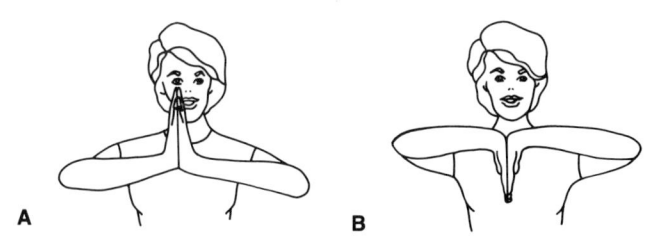

FIG. 18.

Summary

For an exercise program to be of value, it must be designed specifically to meet the needs of a person. Exercises must be performed correctly and on a regular basis. Frequency, rate, and rest periods are important components of the total regimen. The program must be modified to the changes in the patient's condition.

SPLINTS AND BRACES

The purpose of splinting or bracing may include support for weak muscles, minimizing development of deformities or contractures, providing sustained stretching for tight muscles or joints, decreasing extraneous movement, and, in some instances, increasing awareness of the position of the limb in space. It is important to point out that these devices can only serve as adjuncts to other measures. "Function does not flow from the application of inert material, but only function will breed function." Braces and splints must be carefully designed to meet the specific needs of the individual. When braces or splints are applied, it is imperative to examine the limb frequently to insure that no undue pressure occurs over bony prominences and that skin breakdown is avoided. Although there have been considerable changes in the materials used and the methods of fabricating splints and braces, they still tend to add weight, and the movement permitted while wearing a brace is different from "normal" physiological motion. One needs to weigh carefully the potential benefits and risks of these devices.

9

Making Everyday Activities Easier

Kate Robbins and Brian Rosenthal

Multiple sclerosis (MS) often results in difficulty walking and in using the arms and hands because of weakness, spasticity, and loss of coordination. Visual and sensory difficulties may also occur. These do not necessarily occur together, nor are they all inevitable. They may occur rather suddenly, last for a while, and then improve; or they may occur slowly with less likelihood of improvement. In either case, there may be a reduction in the ability to walk effectively or to perform adequately the activities we encounter in daily living.

There are many adaptive devices, architectural modifications, and adaptive techniques that make everyday activities easier and safer. The best way to find out which ones can help you is to consult a rehabilitation specialist: a physiatrist, occupational therapist, physical therapist, or rehabilitation nurse. The rehabilitation specialist can evaluate your capabilities and needs and make recommendations that will accommodate fluctuations in your condition.

WALKING AIDS

If you have problems walking, you have probably already arranged your environment to make it easier for you to get around. This may mean having heavy pieces of furniture in your home or workspace placed along common pathways to provide support, or grab bars may have been installed for a secure handhold. Often unsafe, this manner of "furniture walking" works only in your own home and may be inconvenient for other family members. A walking aid such as a cane, forearm crutch, or walker can greatly increase your stability and therefore your mobility (Fig. 1). Which aid offers the greatest security, stability, and safety may require consultation with a rehabilitation specialist, who can also instruct you in the best way for you to walk with the aid, go through doorways, sit down, get up from a chair, enter and leave a car, etc. Realize that the "best" walking aid for you may change just as your multiple sclerosis does.

Maintaining mobility and reducing energy expenditure will be enhanced by one common-sense rule: sit whenever possible; save your energy to walk. You might want to try some of the following to save energy: place chairs in major work areas in your kitchen or office, or bring all the work to one area (perhaps on a wheeled utility cart); arrange major supermarket shopping by phone or go during off hours when there are no long checkout lines.

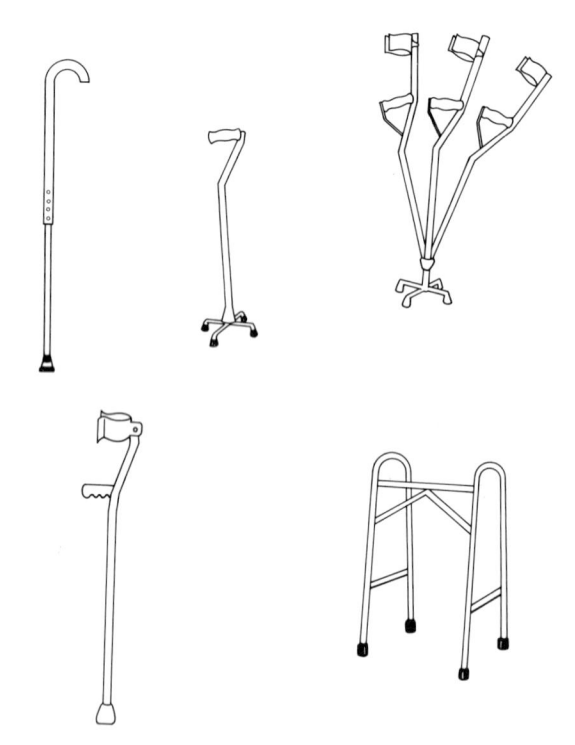

FIG. 1. Walking aids. **Left to right:** straight cane, quad cane, quad cane with swivel-action base, forearm crutch, and walker.

Plan your day based on when you have the most energy and consider what makes you the most tired. In your workplace, could some of the tiring activities be delegated or shared with others? At home, can you enlist the aid of family members or other helpers? For instance: teach the children how to use the washer/dryer.

WHEELCHAIRS

Almost everyone is frightened by the idea of having to use a wheelchair. Visions of confinement and loneliness as well as pity are associated with its use. In fact, this is usually not true. You might consider trying a wheelchair (W/C) when walking with mobility aids becomes too tiring. Even part-time use of a W/C often increases your mobility and sense of freedom, especially if your legs are weaker than your arms.

The choice of the proper chair is important (Fig. 2). Not all W/Cs are alike. Unfortunately, most people are relying on a W/C that is the wrong size, too heavy, difficult to maneuver, and downright uncomfortable. To avoid these problems, consider the following list of dos and don'ts when choosing a chair. If you are in doubt do not hesitate to seek the advice of a qualified professional, as this may save you time and heartache (and maybe even bottom ache) as well as money.

Do

1. Consult a rehabilitation specialist to obtain a W/C that will be tailored to your body size, physical capabilities, and life-style. Today, W/Cs are available in many sizes and have many options.
2. Remember the following: comfort must come first; the narrower the better; the simpler the better.
3. Strongly consider a chair with removable armrests. Wheelchairs with fixed arms may not fit under most desks or tables. Transfers are almost always easier if you can take off the armrest and may be essential if you need to use a sliding board.
4. Footrests should also swing away to allow for ease of transfer and maneuverability.
5. For the best "fit," sit in the W/C and check if there is (a) handwidth space between the seat edge and the back of your

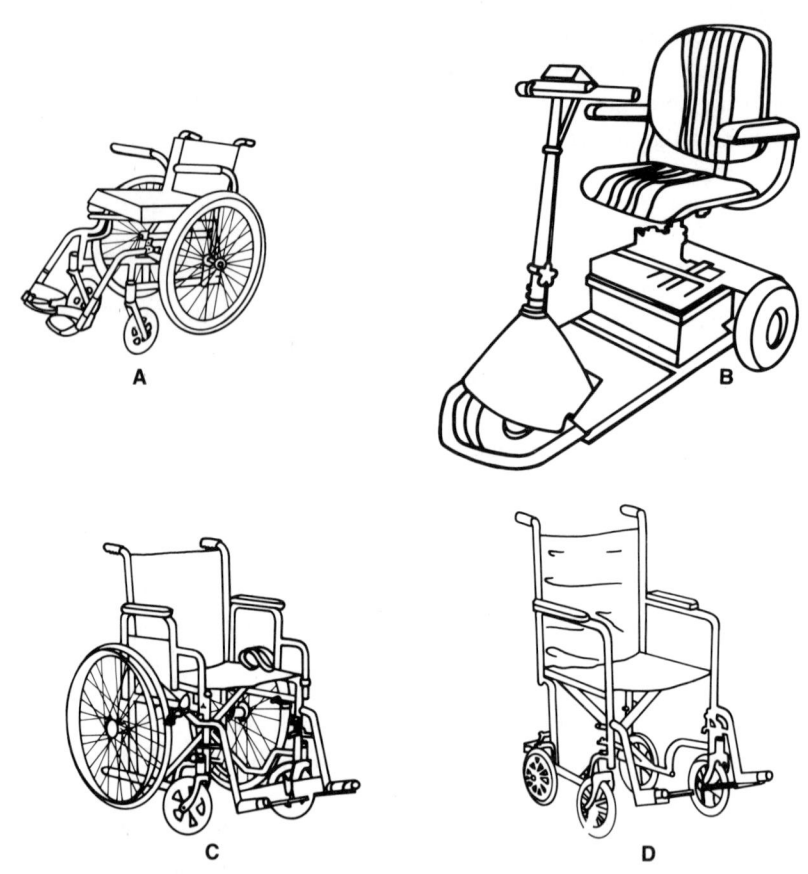

FIG. 2. Different types of wheelchairs. Sports chair **(A)**, scooter **(B)**, standard wheelchair **(C)**, and chair with small wheels, which must be pushed **(D)**.

knee, (b) room for two fingers between your thighs and the W/C sides, (c) a comfortable backrest (top of rest should end at about the middle of your shoulder blades), (d) that your arms rest comfortably on armrests (are your shoulders pushed too high or sagging down?), and (e) that your thighs are parallel to the floor.

Don't

1. Buy a wheelchair from some one else. (It's probably not right for you, and your insurance won't help pay for it.)
2. Order accessories that you don't need. Fancier isn't better.

EVERYDAY ACTIVITIES   113

   3. Use a chair that is broken. Torn seats, broken spokes, split tires, etc. are dangerous for you as well as those who help you.
   4. Use a chair with worn or missing brakes. It is no less dangerous than worn brakes on an automobile.
   5. Allow anyone else to use (or play with) your W/C. A W/C is not a toy, and when it's broken you will suffer until repairs are made.

A seat cushion is not considered an accessory. New cushion material and designs are continually being developed by manufacturers and tested at rehabilitation centers. (That spare throw pillow you have lying around the house is not adequate.) A rehabilitation specialist will consider your weight and body structure in helping you choose the proper cushion or combination of cushions for good posture and stability, prevention of skin breakdown, ease in transfers, and comfort. The vinyl cover used to protect cushions from moisture may be "sticky" and uncomfortable, especially in warm weather. A thick terry towel wrapped around the vinyl, or sewn to fit over the vinyl cover, will help.

Motorized W/Cs with the motor and batteries mounted underneath are similar in appearance to manual wheelchairs. Some manual wheelchairs can even be converted to the motorized variety. Control boxes are placed near the armrest for hand control. Adaptations for chin or breath (sip and puff) control can also be made for the very few extremely disabled. Before purchasing a motorized W/C, it is best to evaluate your ability with the various controls at a rehabilitation center. Motorized W/Cs are very expensive. After removing the batteries, some can be folded for car or plane travel, but they are much heavier than manual W/Cs and require meticulous maintenance.

An increasingly popular alternative to motorized W/Cs are the less-expensive motorized scooters. A scooter operator should have good sitting stability and be able to reach forward with at least one arm and hand to steer and operate the control levers. Advantages of the scooter compared to the W/C are narrower width, swivel seat, and a sportier look. Choose a scooter that has removable armrests and will accommodate a seat cushion. Though motorized scooters can be disassembled for transportation, and lifts have been designed to place the heavier parts in a car, you may still need some help getting the scooter in and out of the car. As with a motorized W/C, it is best to try the various scooters before purchase.

Two distinct types of W/C deserve special attention here. One that is intended to be pushed by a companion has four small wheels. This chair is very narrow and folds compactly, making it easy to maneuver in restaurants, theaters, and other crowded areas; the armrests are fixed, so standing is required when getting in and out of the chair. Remember that you cannot maneuver this chair yourself; someone must push you.

Another is the so-called sports W/C. Many find this W/C easier to maneuver and, because in some models the large rear wheels are removable, easier to transport in a car. For some, this model W/C does not offer enough sitting stability.

WHEN DOORWAYS AND STEPS ARE A PROBLEM

Replacing door hinges with offset hinges will increase the opening 1.5 to 2 inches because the door will swing completely out of the opening. Door saddles (a raised strip of wood or marble where the floors of two rooms or a hallway and a room meet) should be removed and the space between the two floors made level if the saddle interferes with mobility.

A few steps can be ramped if there is room. For every inch in step height, the ramp should be 10 to 12 inches long for a person in a wheelchair to be able to push up the ramp. A platform (5 feet × 5 feet is recommended) at the top of the ramp will enable a person in a wheelchair to unlock and open a door. Mechanical devices such as porch lifts lower a wheelchair on a platform from the porch to street level; in the house, stair lifts carry a seated person up and down a straight or curved flight of stairs. These are expensive and can break down. Whenever possible, a single-level dwelling should be sought.

CAR HAND CONTROLS

Car hand controls have given many people the freedom to drive wherever they wish despite weakness in their legs. If you have good vision and hand function, hand controls can be installed in cars with automatic transmissions. This enables you to operate the brake and gas pedal safely through mechanical attachments. The installation does not interfere with foot operation, so the car can still be driven by other family members.

GRAB BARS

If you have difficulty walking, you may want or need the additional security of grab bars attached to the wall or a lifeguard rail attached to the tub. Grab bars are tubular stainless steel sections mounted into wall support studs. Some are vinyl covered for better grip and less heat absorption.

Grab bars can be mounted in any configuration: horizontal, vertical, diagonal, L-shaped, etc. A space the width of a clenched fist should exist between the grab bar and the wall to permit quick release and regrasp of the bar. If you are installing the bars yourself, follow the manufacturer's directions exactly; otherwise have them installed professionally. **Never, never use towel racks, soap dishes, door knobs, etc. for support in the bathroom.** These fixtures were not designed to support your body weight. Install a grab bar.

A lifeguard rail is also tubular stainless steel but in the configuration of an inverted U and can be securely attached by suction cups to the tub to provide a sure handhold.

BATHING

This important everyday activity may pose special problems if you have impaired sensation. To avoid burns, do not use your hands to test the water temperature. Rely on an inexpensive thermometer taped to the inside of the tub. Thermometers and thermostats that attach to a shower head are also available. The water temperature should not exceed 100°F.

If getting in and out of the shower or bath is a problem, you may want to consider one of the aids described below (Fig. 3).

Getting to the bottom of the tub and up again is difficult, but if stepping over the tub rim is no problem, then a shower chair used in conjunction with grab bars or a lifeguard rail may be helpful.

116 *EVERYDAY ACTIVITIES*

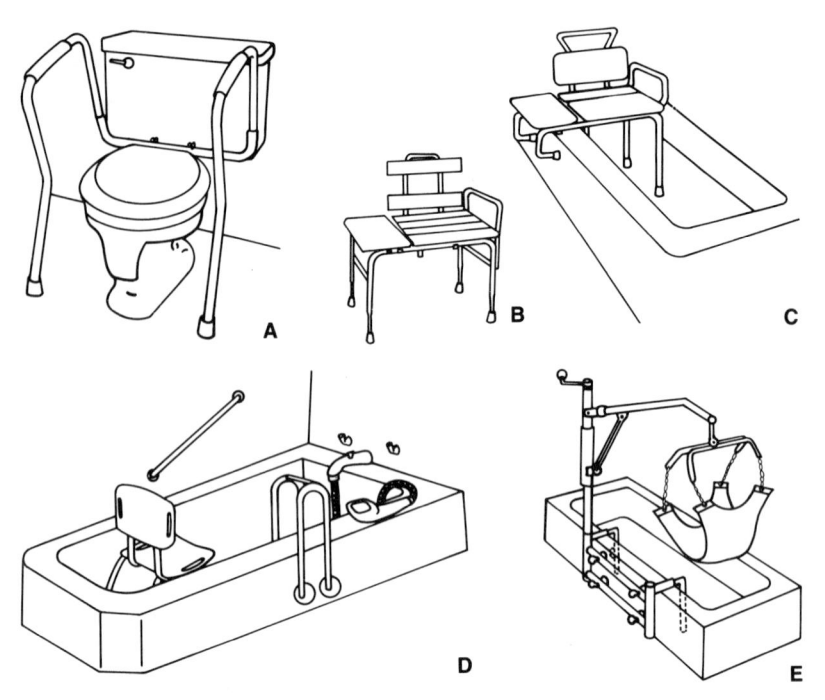

FIG. 3. Bathroom aids. Toilet frame **(A)**, transfer bench **(B)**, bathing bench **(C)**, shower chair, lifeguard rail, diagonal grab bar, and hand-held shower hose **(D)**, and patient lifter and bath attachment **(E)**.

A transfer tub bench is a solid platform that extends across the tub. One with a back support is the safest solution when you cannot safely step over the tub rim. Transferring to the bench involves a sliding transfer from a W/C, then lifting the legs over the tub rim; if walking aids are used, it involves sitting on the bench and then lifting the legs over the rim. An occupational therapist, physical therapist, or other rehabilitation specialist should work with you until you feel secure doing the transfer. Most shower doors do not permit enough room for the transfer tub bench and transferring. Shower doors should be replaced by a shower curtain.

The easiest way to bathe while seated on a transfer tub bench is with a hand held shower hose. A secure mat or nonslip treads are a must in the bathtub.

A much more expensive alternative to the transfer tub bench is the bath lift. Powered by water pressure, this bath seat rises above the tub rim, swivels for transfers, then lowers to the bottom of the tub. Again, a therapist should be consulted to evaluate whether you can safely transfer to the bath lift and independently manage the controlling levers (unfortunately placed behind or beneath the seat).

If you cannot transfer to any type of tub bench, a patient lifter may be attached to the tub rim to lift you from a W/C into the tub (Fig. 4). You may wish to use an inflatable cushion as a backrest

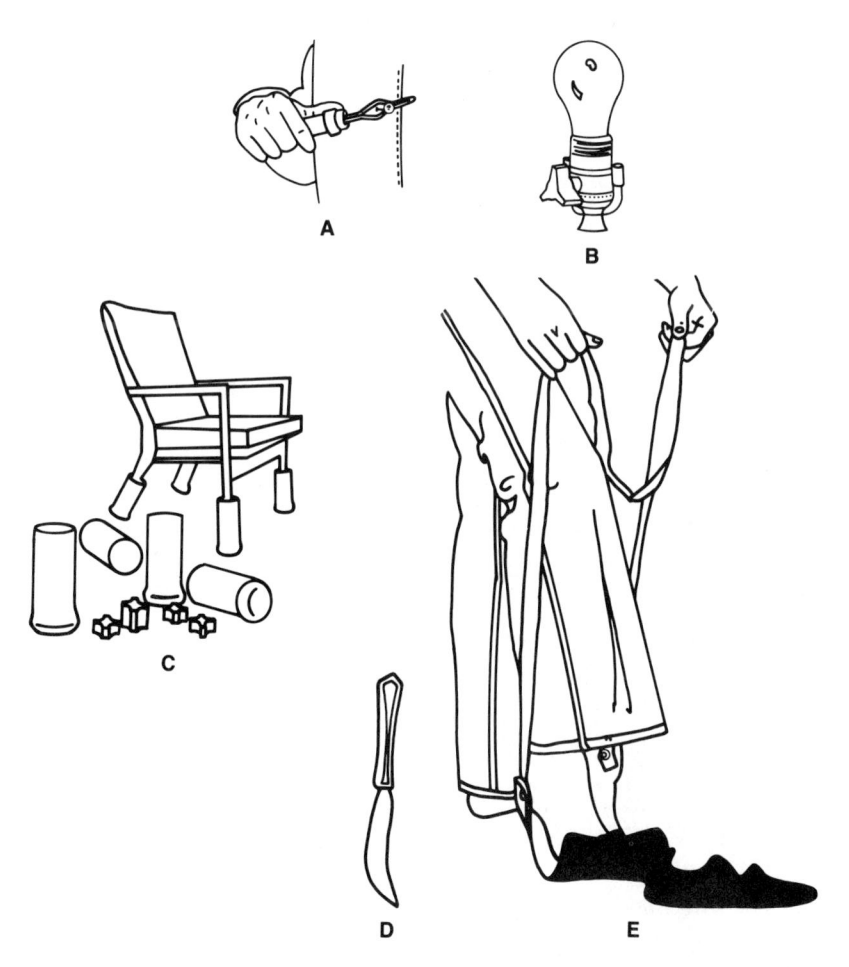

FIG. 4. Useful gadgets. Button aid **(A)**, lamp switch extension lever **(B)**, chair leg extenders **(C)**, rocker knife **(D)**, and sock aid **(E)**.

while soaking. One manufacturer also makes a vinyl tub that is attached to the patient lifter for a tub bath in bed.

Bathing or showering may be made easier by a long-handled sponge (some even hold the soap) to wash hard-to-reach places, a wash mitt (eliminates the need to hold a wash cloth), and a Little Octopus® suction holder (tiny suction cups on both sides of a flat rubber disc firmly hold soap, shampoo bottles, etc. to the tub rim or shower shelf).

TOILETING

The conventional toilet seat is often too low but can be altered with a removable or quickly installed raised toilet seat (also available with a padded seat) to increase the height 4 to 7 inches. If more assistance is needed when lowering to or rising from the toilet seat, grab bars should be placed on the wall alongside the toilet, or an easily installed toilet frame may be used on one or both sides (Fig. 3).

Although a raised toilet seat is the easiest and quickest way to increase the height of the toilet seat, the entire fixture may be raised on a platform, or a wall-hung toilet may be installed. A wall-hung toilet has the additional advantage that it does not take up floor space and permits a closer approach by a W/C.

An electronically powered bidet unit attached to an existing toilet provides an easy way to cleanse yourself after toileting if hand coordination problems make using tissue difficult or if weakness limits arm motion.

USING THE BATHROOM SINK

An open area below the bathroom sink high enough to clear your knees is optimal. To prevent burns, the hot water pipe and drainage pipe **must be insulated.** If you have tremors, a single-lever faucet may be more difficult to control than a faucet operated by two paddle-shaped handles. For convenience, an extra shelf below a high medicine cabinet will hold frequently used items, and a mirror on a flexible or extension arm can be positioned anywhere you need it. If it is impossible

EVERYDAY ACTIVITIES

or very uncomfortable to use the sink in a small bathroom, consider placing toiletry items and a small mirror near the kitchen sink.

SHAMPOOING

Shampooing is probably easiest when showering or bathing with a flexible shower hose. If your hair must be washed while you are confined to bed, an inflatable shampoo basin will support your head in sudsy water and allow water to drain away through a tube to a bedside container.

SHAVING

An electric razor is safest for shaving if you have tremors. Some reduction of tremors may be achieved by stabilizing your head against a headrest, grasping with your free hand the wrist of the hand holding the razor, and keeping your elbows close to your body. A lightweight 1- to 2-lb wrist weight on the hand holding the razor may give additional stability. A razor holder (a strap that attaches the electric razor securely to the palm of the hand) will prevent the razor from accidentally slipping from your grip.

ORAL HYGIENE

A toothbrush with a built-up handle or an electric toothbrush may be easier to handle than a conventional one. If tremors are a problem, try the stabilization techniques suggested above. Toothpaste in a pump dispenser might make things easier.

USING THE KITCHEN

The goal of the functional kitchen is to help you save time and energy. Often the careful selection of appliances, their placement, and the use of kitchen gadgets may lessen the effort involved in meal preparation. If you are lucky enough to have the opportunity to completely redesign your kitchen, a U-shaped or L-shaped kitchen with unbroken counter space is preferable. The major appliances should be placed in the following order: refrigerator, sink, and stove/oven, with counter space between them. This enables you to take food from the refrigerator, wash or prepare it at the sink and counter space, then move it to the stove or oven for cooking or baking.

With a little thought, all food preparation can be done sitting down. A strategically placed sturdy kitchen stool with backrest and footrest, a chair on casters, or a W/C will allow you to cook while seated and thus conserve energy. When a wheelchair or standard-height chair is used, counter space is generally too high for comfortable work; an extra cushion may be all that is necessary to increase the height, but check with your doctor or therapist to make sure your stability in the wheelchair is not at risk with the additional height.

A counter top height of 30 to 32 inches (27 inches for mixing) is best. Determine the most comfortable height for you by working at a few different heights. This can be tested in the training kitchen of a rehabilitation center. If lowering the counter space is not possible, consider a wheeled table, drop-leaf table, or fold-down table hinged to the wall where it could conveniently serve as a work surface. If you are seated at the work surface, you will need knee room underneath. Knee room can sometimes be created under a counter by removing cabinet doors.

Once you have found a comfortable work height, determine how far you can easily reach forward, upward, and downward. Store your most commonly used cookware and foodstuffs within this span of reach.

Like every good cook, organize your cooking utensils according to their use and your need: salad items together between the refrigerator and sink, mixing bowls and baking pans together near the oven, skillet near the stove, and tea kettle near the sink. Duplicate your most frequently used items (measuring spoons, small mixing bowl, knife); extra sets will save extra steps. The small cost is worth your energy savings. Items bought in bulk or large containers may be easier to manage when they are transferred to smaller canisters. Generally, lightweight canisters are better if you have weakness; heavy canisters are better if you have tremors.

Maximize Storage Space

For your comfort and convenience consider modifying your storage spaces.

Counter Space

A pullout platform at the back of the counter rolls appliances within easy reach. Vertical dividers (for cookie sheets, muffin tins, etc.) can be placed at the back of the counter.

Kitchen Cabinets

A revolving shelf unit (turntable) puts more items within easy reach. An added shelf or pullout basket beneath the upper cabinets utilizes this empty space. To prevent your most commonly used kitchen tools from being pushed out of your reach, simply place large and/or little-used items at the back of the shelf. When lower cabinet doors are removed, open shelf space is created. Drawers or pullout bins can be added. If shelves are removed, sliding racks with hooks to hang such things as pots or cups can be installed. Do not forget that many new small appliances are made to be hung or mounted to add counter space.

Wall Space

Make your walls serve you. Extra shelves, grids, or a pegboard with hooks at a convenient height will utilize wall space.

Closet

Narrow shelves with a lip or guard on the back of the closet door will hold cleaning items or canned goods. (Stronger door hinges will be needed.) For small closets, consider a set of shelves on a dolly that pulls completely out to bring everything within reach. The shelves should have a restraining lip or guard so items do not slip. A mechanical reacher for lightweight items (a pudding box, not a large can of vegetables) can be very helpful.

Sinks and Appliances

Refrigerator

Choose a refrigerator to meet your needs. It is best when the open refrigerator door(s) does not block counter space. This way, food taken from the refrigerator can be placed directly on the counter. If the door blocks the counter space, a wheeled cart is useful for holding the food and can be pushed to the work area where the food is prepared.

There are many styles and sizes of refrigerators. When selecting one, consider the locations of the cooling and freezing compartments. A side-by-side model may offer the best accessibility. A self-defrosting unit will save you a great deal of effort.

Store your heaviest foods within easy reach. Revolving turntable units can be used here too.

Adding shelves in the freezer will prevent stacking too many items, which then become difficult to see and to reach. If the freezer is too deep to reach items in the back, water-filled plastic bottles placed in the back of the freezer will freeze and reduce the energy required to maintain the freezer temperature as well as prevent stored items from being pushed to the back of the freezer beyond reach.

If your refrigerator/freezer does not have an automatic ice cube maker, carrying a half-full ice cube tray to the freezer is easier, as is placing trays in the freezer and filling them with fresh water from a plastic squeeze bottle.

The Sink

A shallow sink with the drain at the rear corner is ideal, as this will give you the most knee room when seated. If your sink is too deep, consider raising it by the use of a custom-fitted wood slat platform or maybe simply turning a dishpan upside down. A rubber mat on the sink bottom reduces breakage. Hot water pipes, the underside of the sink, and the drain should be covered with insulation to prevent burns. If you have decreased sensation in your lower extremities, you might not be aware of these potentially hot surfaces.

A retractable spray hose is useful not only for rinsing dishes in the drying rack but for filling pans with water on the stove or filling pans on the counter and sliding them to the stove. Faucet handles may need an extension for reachability. You may be able to replace them with large paddle-shaped handles (easier to manage with tremors) or a single-lever handle (easier to manage with one hand if your hands are weak). If you are redesigning your kitchen, strongly consider a dishwasher.

Cooking and Baking

A conventional range/oven combination may require the seated individual to cook sideways. Unfortunately, the controls may not be easy to reach, and the broiler may be so low that it is dangerous. To make things easier, arrange a work space to one side and remove lower cabinets to provide knee room. Keep oven racks clean so that baking pans will slide out partway on removal. Use barbecue tongs to reach food in the broiler. If your stove is still not accessible, consider replacing it with a lower self-cleaning oven with a side-opening door or one that opens in front to serve as a shelf. Optimally, burners should be placed in a row to prevent burns while reaching over a hot front burner to one in back. Have these installed at the lowered counter height.

Another less expensive and perhaps the best alternative is to use smaller appliances, such as a self-cleaning toaster-oven/broiler or microwave oven and an immersible electric skillet. An advantage of the microwave oven is that dishes remain cool while the food is being heated. Most recipes can be prepared in these smaller appliances, and they may be much easier to use if you are preparing food for only one or two people. Other appliances that may be useful are a coffee maker, a hot-pot for boiling water, a slow cooker, a mixer, and a blender or food processor.

When choosing an appliance, make sure the controls are easy to

124 *EVERYDAY ACTIVITIES*

reach and to manipulate and that you can disassemble and reassemble the various parts for cleaning. Some controls can be built up by attaching a larger knob or lever for easier grasp. Difficult-to-read temperature settings can sometimes be marked over a larger area of the appliance with bright, heat-resistant paint. Keep only those appliances you use regularly, so storage space is not taken up by little-used items, and meal cleanup does not involve washing every appliance in the kitchen.

The addition of several appliances in the kitchen may draw too much power from the available outlets. An electrician can determine if you need another electrical line to the kitchen and can install a heavy-duty outlet box with extra outlets and a circuit breaker for safety.

Safety Techniques

1. Wear long heat-resistant oven mitts when removing food from the oven.
2. Never lift hot food or liquid across your body.
3. To light a gas burner or oven, place a lighted wooden match near the gas outlet, then turn on the gas. Alternatively, use a flint lighter that creates a spark when the handles are squeezed together (look for this item at camping stores).

Cutting Food

1. A serrated knife is easier to control than one with a straight blade.
2. Use a rocker knife with a curved blade (Fig. 4) or one-handed food chopper if one of your hands is weak.
3. Some food is easier to cut with kitchen shears than with a knife.
4. If you use an electric knife, choose a cordless model.
5. To peel vegetables use an old-fashioned vegetable peeler with two floating blades rather than a knife.

Transferring Hot Liquids and Foods

1. Ladle rather than pour hot liquids from a pan.
2. A baster will remove a small amount of hot liquid.

EVERYDAY ACTIVITIES 125

3. To remove food (vegetables, pasta, etc.) from boiling water, boil the food in a steamer or deep-fry basket, which can be lifted out of the pan.

Frying Food

1. Choose long utensils.
2. Use barbecue tongs to turn food.
3. Wear a flame- and heat-retardant barbecue (or high-school chemistry) apron.

Stabilization Techniques and Adaptive Devices

1. Place a damp cloth or sponge under a bowl to prevent slippage.
2. Double suction-cup holders hold a bowl even more firmly.
3. A cutting board with two nails in the center holds food steady.
4. A pan stabilizer (Fig. 5) attaches to the range by suction cups and limits movement of the pan.
5. A mixing bowl holder holds the bowl for mixing and then tilts for pouring.
6. Kitchen gadgets are available in housewares departments and

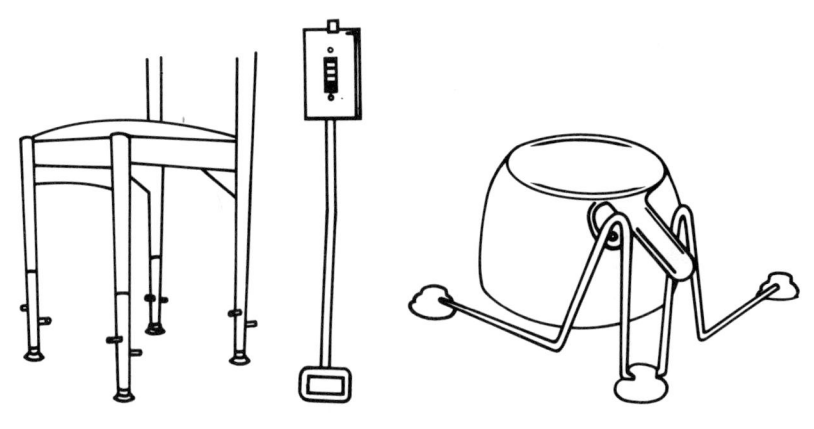

FIG. 5. More useful gadgets. **Left to right:** chair leg extenders, wall light switch extender, and pan stabilizer.

from self-help catalogs. The list is endless; these are just a few that many people have found helpful:
  a. Plastic grater that fits into its own bowl.
  b. Whisk and eggbeaters operated by a downward pushing motion.
  c. One-hand flour sifter with squeeze handle.
  d. Pizza roller for small amounts of pastry dough.
  e. One-hand rolling pin.
  f. Pastry blender (easy to grasp and use with one hand).
  g. Zim jar opener.
  h. Giant pop bottle opener.
  i. Self-wringing sponge mop. (If you are using it from a seated position, saw the handle off at a convenient length, about 30 inches or so.)
  j. Long-handled dust pan.
  k. Plastic washtub on casters.
  l. Cordless, rechargeable, lightweight appliances (mixers, irons, knives).
7. Some aids that may prove helpful when eating are:
  a. Built-up handles to make thin utensils easier to grasp (a foam hair curler placed over the utensil handle may work well).
  b. A rocker knife for one-handed cutting.
  c. A plastic tumbler with lid and holder for a straw or a Vac-u-Flow cup with lid and built-in straw may prevent liquids from spilling. (When drinking hot liquids, use a terry cloth coaster that fits around the bottom of the cup.)
  d. Some people have found that 1- to 2-lb wrist weights help steady tremors when they are eating.

THE BEDROOM

A bedroom that is easy to move around in, where everything is comfortably placed, may require only a little rearranging and few modifications. To make transfers easier, the bed height can be lowered by shortening the legs of the bed frame or raised by using leg extenders or wooden blocks (with at least a 3-inch-deep cutout to hold the leg securely). A backrest or several pillows layered to support the shoulders and head and an over-bed table are useful if you spend much time in bed. (If you use a wheelchair, choose an over-bed table with a base that fits around a wheelchair.) An adjustable bed, manual or motorized, may be the best solution if you are most comfortable in bed. If it is difficult for you to change position in bed, a foam "egg crate" mattress placed directly under the sheet will reduce the pressure, or if you have ever had skin breakdown (pressure sore), your doctor will recommend one of the many other pressure-reducing/pressure-distributing mattresses.

A bedside table to hold water, a telephone, buzzer, or intercom, and other items as well as a good light source should be within convenient reach of the bed. "Gooseneck" holders are available to hold a telephone receiver in one position, and large extensions to fit over both rotary and pushbutton phones make dialing easier. Telephone units with a memory eliminate dialing frequently used numbers. Simple adaptations can also be added to the lighting fixture if it is difficult to use: a knob or curtain ring at the end of a pull cord makes it easier to grasp, a large lamp switch extension lever fits over small lamp switches (Fig. 4), and an extender brings too-high wall switches within reach (Fig. 5). Recently on the market are remote control boxes that enable you to turn on/off a number of electrical devices (such as lights, television, and air conditioner). On/off control switches are also available on extension cords—just be sure the cord is well out of the way (perhaps taped to the baseboard) to prevent tripping over it or becoming entangled in it.

The most comfortable storage height, whether standing or seated, is between shoulder and knee height. If drawers stick, try a silicone spray or refit with glides if possible. If the drawers are difficult to open because two handles are widely spaced, try pulling on a wide ribbon tied between the two handles or replacing them with one large centered handle. A lowered closet rod will accommodate shirts, folded slacks, jackets, skirts, and dresses folded at the waist.

Some aids that may be helpful when dressing are the following:

1. Placing your foot on a stepstool when tying your shoes if you can't reach to the floor.
2. Elastic shoe laces (your feet slip into the shoe without retying)

or Velcro closures (which must be sewn on at a shoe repair shop).
3. A long-handled shoe horn.
4. A button aid that slips through the button hole, attaches around the button, and pulls it through the hole using only one hand (Fig. 4).
5. A stocking aid that holds pantyhose or socks open, allowing you to slip your foot into the sock and pull the sock up (Fig. 4).
6. Velcro to replace difficult to manage hooks and eyes, snaps, zippers, etc.

10

Nursing Care

Nancy J. Holland, Phyllis Wiesel-Levison, and Frances Francabandera

The person with multiple sclerosis (MS) and his or her family may benefit from nursing services in a variety of settings. Although the hospital may be the most familiar place associated with nursing, most MS patients rarely require hospital care. The most likely areas in which the nurse will be encountered include the doctor's office, outpatient clinics or MS Centers, rehabilitation facilities, and the home, through Visiting Nurse or Public Health referrals. In addition to providing direct physical care, the nurse is an educator and interpreter of medical terms, and resource for community services, coordinator of care (liaison with physicians and other health professionals), and an advocate for the patient and family.

One of the nurse's most important functions is to interpret technical terms the MS person and family may hear discussed. Once understood, these medical words are less frightening. The nurse can also explain the disease process and what to expect from it, as well as provide a better understanding about the various symptoms and what causes them, the tests the MS patient sometimes has to undergo, and, finally, the treatments prescribed.

Although the nurse has the potential for providing these services, much of the delivery depends on the inquisitiveness of the patient and his or her family. It is best for the individual and family to approach the problem as a modern consumer would who is buying an appliance or a new car—they are, after all, consumers of health care and should adopt a direct and questioning attitude. When the patient has adopted this attitude, he or she has assumed some control over the situation, which in itself can create a more positive atmosphere.

A team approach to the individual in need of medical help fosters comprehensive care and a holistic view of the patient. This means that he or she is viewed as a unique individual who functions in a particular way within his or her family and the community. This approach can be difficult to maintain given the scope of services that may be required, the number of health care providers involved, and the geographically scattered agencies called on to address assorted needs. The nurse often assumes the role of coordinator of these services.

PHILOSOPHY OF HEALTH CARE

The philosophy of modern health care views health as the optimal level of function and well-being within the possible limitations imposed by a physical or emotional impairment. From this viewpoint, a person with congenital deafness can be healthy, as can a person with MS. For the individual with MS, an important component of health is the absence of disease activity—a remission (disappearance) of symptoms—or stabilization—no further progression of symptoms. However, even when this is not the current situation, health as the highest possible level of well-being is still a goal.

GOOD HEALTH

Implicit in the concept of health is the idea of freedom from illness, which for the MS person means good general health as well as an absence of disease-related complications.

Nutrition

Maintaining good health starts with proper nutrition. There are various aspects of nutrition that are important. It is essential to keep body weight within the proper range for the individual's height and frame. This is a very practical consideration. The MS individual may find it difficult to walk—and with excess weight it becomes even harder.

Transferring from a wheelchair to the toilet or a car becomes a major feat for the obese person. Conversely, the very thin wheelchair-bound person who has insufficient "padding" to protect against pressure and potential skin breakdown (pressure sores) needs to increase caloric intake.

The patient with inadequate nutrition may be more prone to infection, and so a diet of nutritious foods is advised to attain the desired body weight.

Constipation may be a problem that is caused by inadequate fluid intake. In these cases increased bulk and more fluids should be added to the diet. Unprocessed bran is helpful, as are fresh and cooked fruits and vegetables, whole-grain bread, and prune juice.

Urinary tract infections are sometimes a problem for MS patients. Here certain dietary measures can be taken to increase the urinary acidity, which reduces this risk. Cranberry and prune juices promote an acidic urine and are therefore helpful in preventing urinary tract infections. Orange, grapefruit, and tomato juice have components in them that cause the urine to become just the opposite, alkaline, and so should be taken in limited amounts.

As in the general population, some individuals with MS may have other health problems such as diabetes or high blood pressure (hypertension). Diet is of major importance in controlling diabetes, and the physician can recommend a dietary program that includes MS-related needs. Hypertension usually requires salt restriction. When diuretics (drugs to remove excess fluid from the body) are also needed, measures used to manage MS urinary problems may need to be readjusted. The nurse can assist with determining the necessary dietary changes and help the MS person and family with meal planning that follows the individually prescribed diet.

Rest and Exercise

Good health requires an adequate balance between rest and physical activity. The proper balance varies for each individual, one having a need for more rest or sleep than another. The MS person must take care to maintain this delicate balance, since he or she may become easily fatigued. In addition, intolerance of heat and humidity may be a problem. It is believed that greater energy is required to transmit signals in the nervous system past the damaged myelin (the fatty material around the nerve that is damaged or destroyed in MS) than is needed when the nervous system is intact. If this is true, then minimal physical activity may result in a disproportionate energy drain or sense of fatigue. Furthermore, anything that raises the body temperature may heighten this energy loss and/or accentuate any MS symptoms the person is experiencing.

When the MS person is easily fatigued or finds heat sensitivity a problem, exercise must be carefully planned so as not to use up all the individual's energy, leaving little or none for other activities necessary to daily living such as work and socialization.

The visiting nurse or public health nurse agencies can often refer a physical therapist to plan a home program of exercise aimed at maintaining muscle strength and joint mobility while conserving energy for activities of daily living. The most highly recommended exercise is swimming since body temperature is not elevated and buoyancy in the water permits greater movement. Exercise may be done in an air-conditioned room, which controls heat and humidity, so the body does not become overheated.

Rest periods to maximize energy during the day may need to be scheduled. Individuals with MS often have a high energy level during the morning but experience increasing fatigue in the afternoon hours. Recognizing this, a daily schedule can be planned with the more tiring or demanding activities scheduled for the morning hours. For example, the housewife may choose to shop early in the day when stores are less crowded and her energy level is higher. Light household chores and dinner preparation can then be done at a more leisurely pace in the afternoon, with a brief rest period or nap if needed. When low energy or a pattern of easy exhaustion is encountered, alternating activity with rest periods will usually improve overall function.

Non-Exercise-Related Body Temperature Elevation

Any individual's body temperature may increase when struck by "flu," a sore throat, or other infection. Even with a slight elevation, the person with MS may find that weakness worsens to the extent that a person who is normally ambulatory may not be able to walk. Fortunately, this worsening of symptoms is usually temporary (pseudoexacerbation), as it is after excessive exercise. However, the doctor or nurse should always be called when this occurs.

Corrective measures for this weakening effect are aimed at identifying and eliminating the cause of the fever when possible, as with a urinary tract or other infection, and at reducing the body temperature to normal.

The temperature may be reduced by taking aspirin or acetaminophen (Tylenol) every 4 hours along with drinking cool fluids. The patient's temperature should be checked every 4 to 6 hours to make sure it is being lowered.

If the infection is severe (for instance if there is a possible severe urinary tract infection, pneumonia, or an infected pressure sore), or if the person is already very ill, the doctor may recommend hospitalization.

Hot baths or showers, steam from a hot stove or iron, or prolonged exposure to the sun may also temporarily elevate the body temperature. The first effect from this elevated body temperature may show up as slight blurring of the vision or a general feeling of weakness.

When a person with MS realizes that there is a problem with heat intolerance (from any source), he or she should minimize situations in which the body becomes overheated.

SYMPTOMS DIRECTLY RELATED TO MS

The person with MS can, at any given time, experience symptoms of the disease. Because this is so, it is well to recognize the symptoms and to know how to relieve them.

A symptom is a perceptible change in the body or its functions that indicates disease. Symptoms of MS vary in severity, duration, and effect on the individual's daily function. Their significance in terms of the course of the disease and in terms of the individual's response to therapy also is quite different from one patient to another. Given the diversity of potential symptoms, the person with MS may find it difficult to sort out which symptoms are MS related and which are not. In this situation the nurse or physician should be contacted to help resolve the question and to prescribe symptomatic treatment when available. Moreover, such a change may signify a point at which more aggressive therapy should be considered.

Sensory symptoms—numbness, tingling, a sense of constriction as if a tight band had been applied, and vague, peculiar skin sensations—tend to be temporary. They may "come and go" for a number of months. Some sensory disturbances are more troubling, such as burning or pain along the course of a nerve. These are also temporary and may be controlled by medication such as carbamazepine (Tegretol), phenytoin sodium (Dilantin), or amitriptyline (Elavil). Although sensory symptoms may cause discomfort, they are considered benign in that they do not affect the overall prognosis of MS.

Visual symptoms such as blurring, pain in the eye, or "blind spots" also tend to be temporary and do not signify a serious course of MS. These symptoms may be alleviated more rapidly if steroids are administered, and so a short course of oral prednisone or dexamethasone (Decadron) is sometimes prescribed by the physician.

Motor symptoms are those that interfere with movement. In the MS patient these are seen most frequently as leg weakness. Coordination problems include imbalance while walking, involuntary hand movements, and jumping of the eyes. Although motor and coordination symptoms are often resistant to treatment, some therapies are available. These are described in Chapter 8.

Symptoms caused by bladder or bowel dysfunction should be reported to the doctor, who can prescribe various measures to relieve them (see Chapter 11). A small percentage of patients with advanced MS have more serious symptoms, which are discussed later in this chapter.

When concern about a symptom is present, the MS person or family should contact the nurse, who can then help determine the proper course of action to pursue. This may be a visit to the doctor or local emergency room or simply reassurance that no action is needed. Again, the nurse's role is to provide information for better understanding of the disease and its manifestations.

SKIN PROTECTION

A person's skin condition is rarely a topic for conversation. For the MS person with advanced disease, however, it is of prime importance to understand how the skin acts as a protective agent, how to recognize and prevent potential problems, and the relevance of good hygiene and a well-balanced diet.

Skin constitutes the outer covering of the entire body. There are several layers of this covering, which protect body tissues from outside harm. Any break in the skin through which bacteria may enter is a potential source of infection. Such breaks may be caused by irritation or by rubbing a particular area for prolonged periods. In addition, prolonged contact with moisture, as may occur with urinary leakage, may also precipitate skin breakdown. However, the major threat for susceptible MS patients is skin breakdown caused by pressure.

People with MS who have sensory deficits are candidates for skin breakdown, since signals indicating too much pressure are not felt (or only slightly so). Pressure on a particular body area for any length of time, without the person moving or changing position to reduce the pressure, decreases the blood flow to that spot. This reduces the oxygen and nutrients necessary for tissue health. If an area lacks these components for a long period of time, the tissue may die (necrosis). This process may begin after only an hour of continuous pressure and is much more difficult to reverse than to prevent.

The result of such reduced circulation is a pressure sore (also known as a bedsore or a decubitus ulcer). It usually occurs over bony prominences (sacrum, ankles, elbows) and other pressure points (heels). The earliest sign of this sore is a reddened area that progresses to a superficial skin blister, which subsequently opens. Alternatively, the sore may start as a blackened, soft area under the skin. Fluid may ooze from the sore, and the affected area may increase in width and depth. Once the problem is recognized, treatment should be initiated. Specific treatment is discussed later in this section.

Pressure sores may also be caused by a device such as a leg or hand brace that is improperly fitted or poorly padded. They can appear on the person confined to a wheelchair or one who is sitting all day in an office. It is extremely important to keep in mind that when there is a decrease in sensation one will not feel the damaging pressure, and so the sore will be discovered only after harmful effects have occurred. The key to good skin care is thus awareness and prevention.

If the wheelchair-bound person is able to stand, he should do so every hour for about 1 to 3 minutes. An excellent way to relieve pressure on the sacrum and tuberosities (buttocks) is to lock the wheelchair, hold onto its sides or to a table in front of the wheelchair, and then stand. The person unable to stand may lock the chair and do push-ups by grasping the arms of the chair. Both of these exercises relieve pressure on the buttocks and sacrum and allow improved blood flow to that area. A good seat cushion is an essential preventative item for the wheelchair-bound person.

Swelling and/or discoloration of the ankles and feet usually indicates poor circulation in the lower extremities. Blood flow from the feet and legs is normally aided by pumping action of the calf muscles, and so decreased activity of the leg muscles results in an accumulation of fluid. This may predispose to skin breakdown. For this reason the wheelchair-bound person should occasionally elevate his or her legs on the wheelchair foot rests or place them on a chair or sofa to reduce swelling. Actively or passively moving the legs will also help circulation, as will having the legs raised and lowered by another person. Support stockings may also be helpful, as will an exercise called the "ankle pump." A belt (or towel) is held with an end in either hand. Each foot (sequentially) is placed in the center of the belt. By pulling, then releasing the ends of the belt, the foot is alternately flexed and extended. This "pumping" action aids in returning fluid collected in the foot to the body's circulation.

Severely disabled people with MS may easily develop pressure sores. In order to avoid this, the bed-ridden MS person should do additional exercises.

Turn from side to side or onto the abdomen every 2 hours, even during the night. The MS person may be able to turn independently; if not, he or she may help the care giver by grasping the side rails and pulling the body over or by using an overhead trapeze (attached to the bed). Pillows should be positioned in strategic places (a) for comfort, (b) to prevent any unintentional change in position, and (c) to avoid pressure over a bony prominence. When lying on the side, one pillow is placed between the lower legs to separate the knees and ankles, and one behind the back to provide support. After turning, massage the area that has been lain on with a skin lotion or cream to help restore circulation. Creased sheets should also be smoothed at this time.

An air or water mattress, gel foam mattress, and sheepskin heel and elbow protectors are also useful measures for preventing pressure sores. In addition, a bath every other day (in bed or tub) is needed, as is good care of the nails. These should be cut to prevent the patient from accidently scratching and breaking the skin. Care should be taken when cutting toenails to reduce trauma and infection. Nails should be cut straight across and not too short. The services of a podiatrist may be required in some cases. It is also extremely important to ensure adequate nutrition to keep the body tissues healthy and less prone to breakdown.

Prevention of skin breakdown is an important goal because the consequences of pressure sores are significant. When a sore occurs:

1. Long periods of immobility are required to promote healing, as the absence of pressure and exposure to the air are needed for healing.
2. Tissue damage can extend to underlying skeletal structures, resulting in bone infection (osteomyelitis), which tends to be chronic and poorly controlled.
3. Extensive muscle/skin grafting may be needed because of the generally poor blood circulation to areas of potential skin breakdown. (Poor circulation interferes with the healing process.)
4. Infection rapidly develops after the skin breaks down, and damage easily occurs to the tissues underneath. This may proceed to "blood poisoning" (septicemia) and may be life-threatening.

Treatment of Pressure Sores

At the first sign that a pressure sore is forming, measures should be initiated to prevent worsening. If an area on the body is excessively red, massage it with a skin lotion and change the individual's position. If there is a small break in the skin, the area must be kept clean, dry, and without pressure. The first step is to cleanse the affected skin with povidone iodine (Betadine) solution, a brown antiseptic that may stain linens but is readily removed from the skin with soap and water. Betadine is applied by saturating a gauze pad with the solution and then dabbing the area of skin breakdown. This will cleanse the area, deter infection, and help dry the sore. It is not necessary to place a bandage or gauze pad on the area unless the person will be sitting on the sore for any length of time or it is in an area where there may be contact with feces. A blow-type hair dryer may be used to dry the sore in conjunction with the Betadine. If the dryer is used, blow warm (not hot) air on the sore at a distance of approximately 10 inches. A topical powder, thymol iodide, may be lightly dusted over the site to dry the sore further and avoid infection. Vaseline or other lubricating creams should be avoided at this time, although these may be helpful if the skin has not yet broken.

The nurse should be notified when any skin breakdown is observed. She or he will evaluate the area and advise the patient or caregiver about the appropriate treatment. In some situations a small piece of gauze may be needed to keep skin folds separated, preventing the area from closing on the surface until the underlying tissues have healed. If dead (necrotic) tissue is present, it may need to be gradually cleared away by applying a special enzyme ointment. In some cases the sore seems to be superficial even though the actual damage has progressed to some depth or infection has already started. The nurse may advise immediate examination by a physician and in any event will inform him or her about the status of the pressure sore. The nurse should then continue to monitor the condition of the pressure sore until healing has taken place. She/he will recommend and help to obtain whatever supplies are needed for care. These may include new waterproof dressings, such as DuoDerm or Opsite, which promote healing.

In all cases, pressure must be kept off the affected area. Exposure to the air is also advised as much as possible. When the sore is located on or near the buttocks, the person will be required to remain in bed and off the sore for long periods each day. This may be distressing to the individual who is normally active, but it is essential if more serious, even life-threatening injury is to be avoided.

If the decubitus continues to worsen (becomes wider, deeper, changes color to black, or drains blood, clear fluid, or pus), more aggressive treatment may be required that calls for hospitalization. During this time, the wound may be cleansed in a whirlpool-type bath (Hubbard tank) in which most of the body is immersed. This also helps to improve circulation to the impaired tissues. If the person cannot control urinary flow, a Foley catheter may be inserted to keep the wound dry and promote healing. If the sore has become infected, antibiotics are likely to be administered to prevent a more serious infection from developing.

This is often sufficient treatment to help heal the wound. While in the hospital the MS person may be placed on a special bed.

Recently, a new type of bed to promote pressure sore healing has become available—the Clinitron. This unit is composed of tiny silicone balls in constant motion to provide a floatation effect. This is primarily designed for hospital use, but can be rented for the home. The patient does not require turning, which reduces stress on the MS person and caregiver as well.

A pressure sore rarely requires surgery to close it, but if all else fails this may be recommended. Dead tissue may need to be removed before healing can take place. Circulation is poor in areas where pressure sores usually form, and so it may be necessary to have a skin or muscle graft from an area that has a good blood supply. The area where skin has been removed generally heals without any further difficulty, as does the grafted area.

PASSIVE EXERCISE

Some individuals with MS cannot move one or more of their arms or legs because of weakness, incoordination, or spasticity (muscle stiffness or tightness). When this situation exists, the limb(s) must be passively exercised, either by the MS person or someone else, in order to maintain full movement of that joint (elbow, wrist, knee, ankle). The arm or leg is moved through all the positions that would be possible with a normal limb. All joints need to be moved. In the case of an affected arm, the shoulder, elbow, wrist, and fingers should be manipulated; for the leg it is the hip, knee, ankle, and toes. These exercises, called passive range of motion (PROM), should be done at least twice a day. Bathing and dressing are convenient times for this.

The purpose of the PROM exercises is to maintain full joint mobility, thereby avoiding painful and potentially dangerous contractures. A contracture is a "frozen joint" in which permanent changes in the joint prohibit return of movement. If contracture occurs, surgical correction is needed for mobility to be restored. The contracture interferes with activities of daily living, such as dressing. For example, it is difficult to put on a shirt or jacket if no movement in the shoulder is possible. When the MS person tries to move the frozen joint, he experiences severe pain. Furthermore, contracture means that skin surfaces are continuously in contact, which causes irritation, often resulting in skin breakdown with ulceration. Hygiene is also impaired by the joint immobility.

When spasticity contributes to limitation of movement, the extremity should be gently stretched. Most often the patient holds the leg or arm in a bent (flexed) position. It then needs to be slowly straightened (extended) in order to mobilize the joint.

It is important to keep the body and extremities moving so the circulation is maintained as well as to prevent contractures and pressure sores. Turning from side to side and sitting up in a chair help circulate the blood (oxygen and essential nutrients) throughout the body. This also avoids fluid collection in the lungs and so minimizes the possibility of lung congestion, which may lead to pneumonia. Body movement also reduces the rate at which calcium is lost from the bones, thereby helping to decrease the incidence of stone formation in the urinary system.

It is apparent that the benefits of getting the usually bedridden person into a chair are numerous. The change of position increases comfort, facilitates eating and drinking, and increases the self-esteem of the person. To be able to sit up and be a part of family activities is a wonderful feeling and reduces the sense of isolation.

If needed, the very disabled person can be gotten out of bed by the use of a Hoyer lift or Trans-Aid. These are hydraulic devices operated with very little effort on the part of the caregiver. Tub bathing may be accomplished at this time, as the use of the hydraulic lift makes the task easier (see Chapter 9). Bathing is very refreshing for the patient and maintains good body hygiene. Change of bedding is also done with greater ease while the person is out of bed. Wet or even creased sheets cause discomfort and may contribute to skin breakdown.

The various kinds of passive exercise that may be needed, depending on the MS patient's particular situation, are all useful in promoting comfort and mobility as well as preventing illness caused by complications. The nurse can advise the patient and/or caregiver in the home when the need for passive exercise has been identified.

Correction of Contractures

When joint mobility has become limited, it is necessary to identify if a contracture or merely a stiff joint is present.

A physician who specializes in rehabilitation (physiatrist) may make this determination by physical examination. In some cases the patient may require examination while under general anesthesia (in the hospital) so that an accurate diagnosis can be made.

If a contracture is present, surgical correction is necessary. When joint stiffness results from severely spastic muscles, a nerve block (injection of phenol into the nerve) may be necessary to relax the muscles and permit return of joint mobility. Whichever joint condition is present, a course of physical therapy is needed after the corrective measures in order to maximize restored joint mobility.

SAFETY MEASURES

One must be safe in his own environment in order to prevent unforeseen complications that may result from accidents or injuries. For the person with decreased sensation, special care is in order. For instance, the temperature of bath water must be checked with a thermometer or by the unaffected arm or leg. Otherwise scalding and serious burns may result because of the affected individual's diminished perception of extreme heat.

Caution is also needed in the kitchen or when smoking cigarettes. Padded potholder mitts should be used for removing pots from the stove and baking dishes from the oven. Hot water bottles and heating pads should be avoided unless their use is directly supervised by an unimpaired individual.

Decreased sensory perception can also result in frostbite during cold weather or when storing food in a freezer. Warm clothing, including gloves, should be worn during frigid weather, and oven mitts should be used when handling frozen food for any length of time.

Shoes need to be properly fitted, as blisters can quickly develop without notice when sensation in the feet is impaired.

Accidental falls in the home are another potential danger. Throw rugs should be removed and grab bars installed where needed, as in the bathroom. The MS person should use some mobility aid—whether it is a cane, crutch, walker, or wheelchair—when appropriate. Three or more falls within a month suggest that the proper device is not being used or that the person needs additional training with the particular device.

These and other safety measures can be discussed with the nurse. When a particular problem area is identified, the nurse may refer an occupational or physical therapist for more extensive evaluation and recommendations. More detailed information on safety measures in the home is provided in Chapter 9.

The patient with urinary problems may have another source of potential injury—the catheter that stays inside the bladder (Foley catheter). This catheter is inserted through the urinary opening and is held in place by a small balloon inflated within the bladder. A sudden tug on the catheter may forcibly withdraw it from the bladder, causing internal injury as the inflated balloon exits from the body. This can be avoided by taping the catheter to the upper thigh of the female patient or to lower abdomen of the male patient using hypoallergenic tape.

DEALING WITH SWALLOWING DIFFICULTY

Impaired swallowing is a direct result of advanced MS and is not treatable by any currently known medical therapy. Mild dysfunction may be dealt with by dietary modifications aimed at maintaining adequate nutrition and preventing aspiration pneumonia. This complication occurs when food or fluid goes into the lungs rather than the stomach.

Fluids are frequently difficult to swallow, and so thicker forms such as milkshakes, gelatin, applesauce, pudding, or sherbet may be eaten instead. Food that crumbles (toast, cake, potato chips) should be avoided. Small frequent meals are generally better tolerated than large meals, and soft food is more easily swallowed than solid food, which requires extensive chewing.

When swallowing is impaired to the extent that it is no longer safe to take food by mouth, a surgical procedure will be needed to create an alternate route for food and fluid intake. The two most common procedures are gastrostomy and esophagostomy.

With a gastrostomy, an opening is created in the stomach that is accessible through a tube in the abdomen. The tube is then changed by the nurse or physician every 4 to 6 months. A gauze pad is cut from one edge to its center, placed around the gastrostomy tube, and held there by hypoallergenic tape. In some cases special skin care is needed, as when gastric juices irritate the skin or scar tissue develops. This should be discussed with the nurse.

An esophagostomy is an opening made in the esophagus (the passageway that connects the mouth to the stomach) with access through an opening in the neck. Unlike the gastrostomy, the tube is inserted prior to each feeding, and skin problems are minimal because of the distance from the irritating gastric juices. Blenderized food and fluids are easily "fed" through either the gastrostomy or esophagostomy. Furthermore, the route for normal swallowing remains intact so that small amounts of desired foods may be taken by mouth to provide pleasure through the sense of taste.

OTHER COMPLICATIONS

Other complications may occur, such as pneumonia, but treatment is standard and not specific for MS. Individuals with advanced MS will require care in many or all activities of daily living. These measures are dealt with earlier in this and other chapters.

REHABILITATION

Rehabilitation is defined in *Stedman's Medical Dictionary* as "restoration, following disease, illness, or injury, of ability to function in a normal or near normal manner." In a broader view, rehabilitation includes all efforts to achieve optimal function in activities of daily living, within given limitations of the disease or disability. Many health professionals are involved in rehabilitation, notably physical and occupational therapists, rehabilitation counselors, nurses, social workers, and physicians who specialize in this field (physiatrists). All of these people are concerned with improving the patient's level of function and developing adaptive strategies to maximize the potential of each individual. The development of adaptive strategies is a helpful concept, as rehabilitation is a carefully formulated and continuously revised plan of action. For the person with MS, this ongoing readjustment of goals and activities is essential, although very difficult. What is possible and desirable? This is the major question that must be answered before any rehabilitation effort is undertaken.

OVERCOMING FATIGUE

Determining the most suitable balance of rest and activity/exercise is the initial challenge in reducing easy fatigue as a disability. Other measures can also be advantageous, particularly those that reduce the amount of energy expended in mobility (getting from one place to another).

Most people with MS are ambulatory; some need no help whatsoever, whereas others require assistance. Assistive devices or techniques vary from holding onto walls (wall walking) or onto another person for support to using a cane, crutches, or walker for stability. It is often a slow and painful process to accept an assistive device, as it is first necessary to acknowledge the loss of function. The goal is to view the mobility aid as an asset that expands the scope of possible activities and promotes safety from potentially serious falls rather than as a symbol of disease progression. It is important to recognize that a sense of loss and sadness is bound to accompany increased difficulty in walking, while at the same time being able to accept the value of adopting whatever mobility aid is indicated.

For the struggling ambulatory person, a motorized chair such as a Scooter or Amigo is recommended. These vehicles are smaller than wheelchairs, easily maneuvered, and battery operated. They resemble golf carts, and the components are easily taken apart so they can be transported in the trunk of a car. Sometimes it takes such strenuous efforts just to reach one's destination that the MS person has no energy left for what he set out to do. This struggle can be overcome with these motorized aids, which leave the person with enough energy to accomplish other tasks.

SUMMARY

For the person with MS, sickness—or deviation from general good health—occurs when disease-related complications have developed or when the MS progresses to an advanced, severely debilitating state. As with the focus on the prevention of illness, nursing care falls within the primary objective of health promotion. The treatment of complications is aimed at restoring the person with MS to his or her condition of health prior to the particular difficulty. When MS has progressed to an advanced state, the general goal remains the promotion of health to the optimal level possible within the disease limitations. This concept may be disconcerting for those who have trouble thinking of MS and health together. However, this orientation strives for a positive approach regarding what can be done rather than a negative or hopeless outlook toward the person with MS who is sick because of primary or secondary effects of the disease.

Nursing care is administered not only by the professional nurse but by family members and other caregivers who strive to meet the physical and emotional needs of the person with MS. Although serious problems may be encountered, successful management of MS-related problems can be achieved by the cooperation of the patient, the family, and the person providing nursing care services.

11

Bladder and Bowel Management

Nancy J. Holland and Frances Francabandera

Urinary symptoms are common in multiple sclerosis (MS), with as many as 80% of individuals affected at some time during the course of the disease. Bowel problems, especially constipation, also occur frequently. Symptoms in both of these areas are distressing and may interfere with personal, social, and vocational activities. Symptoms of bladder and bowel disorders, their meaning, and their treatment are discussed in this chapter. Understanding normal function, being able to relate symptoms to the actual physical impairment, and being aware of what can be expected from various treatments will help you identify problems and indications for seeking professional help. It will also help you to participate in your own bladder and bowel management.

DISORDERS OF URINARY FUNCTION

The individual with MS has a good chance of achieving average life expectancy if complications are avoided or minimized. Recurrent urinary tract infection, with its potential for kidney damage, is a major complication and presents an impediment to good health and longevity. The need to urinate frequently and suddenly without warning, and the loss of urinary control, inhibit socialization, interfere with job performance, and cause embarrassment in intimate circumstances (such as sexual activity). Feelings of self-esteem and enthusiasm to pursue rewarding experiences may be greatly diminished.

The hopeful aspect for persons with urinary disorders is that serious complications can be prevented and distressing symptoms relieved. However, some individuals become accustomed to these disorders, and so they need to be reminded that dysfunction exists and be reassured that improvement is possible. Some ways that symptoms are rationalized are: "I wet myself because (a) the front door key stuck; (b) we had to stop for a red light; (c) I had coffee that morning; (d) my kids tie up the bathroom." These excuses might be a reasonable way of dealing with an irreversible problem—but fortunately, bladder symptoms can be relieved. Acknowledgment that a problem exists is the first step and should be considered by anyone with a diagnosis of MS.

NORMAL BLADDER FUNCTION

A person with normal bladder function passes urine only four to six times within a 24-hr period. Urination can be postponed until it is convenient, allowing uninterrupted sleep and the avoidance of "accidental urination."

The urinary bladder stores urine, which is continuously produced by the kidneys and carried to the bladder through two small tubes called ureters (Fig. 1). When about 200 milliliters (ml), which is slightly less than a cup, has accumulated, the individual usually becomes aware of urine in the bladder. Contractions of the bladder, signaling a desire to urinate, are inhibited by the nervous system until 300 to 500 ml (roughly 1 to 2 cups) has collected. At this point, urination (also called voiding) is voluntarily initiated. For voiding to occur, the bladder contracts to expel urine through a thin tube called the urethra. At the same time, a valve-like muscle (the sphincter) in the urethra relaxes so the urine can easily pass. Thus, when an adequate amount of urine is present, the bladder contracts, expelling all of the urine, and the sphincter relaxes, allowing the urine to flow out of the body. This all occurs automatically; but as bladder fullness can be sensed by the individual, emptying can be postponed by voluntarily contracting the sphincter until a more convenient time for voiding.

PROBLEMS IN URINARY FUNCTION

Bladder dysfunction in MS is associated with spinal cord disease and is referred to as *neurogenic bladder*. It may produce the following symptoms:

1. *Urgency.* Once the desire to void is experienced, urination cannot be postponed until convenient. A toilet must always be in close proximity.
2. *Frequency.* The person must void more frequently than every 2 to 3 hours.
3. *Hesitancy.* Once at the toilet, the individual sometimes has difficulty initiating the flow of urine. This may occur despite the sense of "urgency."
4. *Incontinence or enuresis.* Passage of urine occurs before the

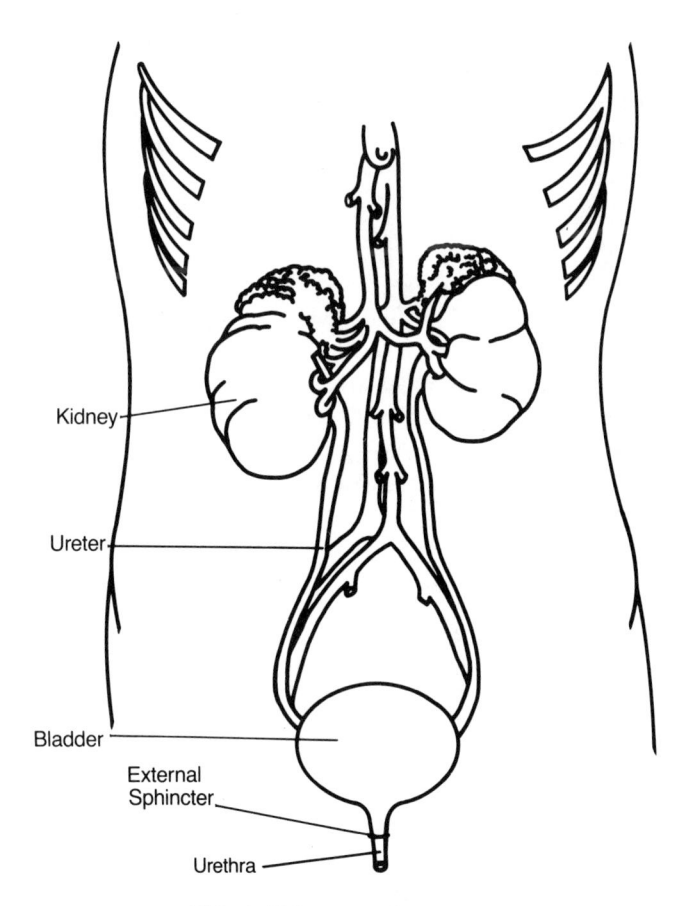

FIG. 1. Urinary tract anatomy.

toilet is reached (accidents). Loss of urinary control during sleep is called nocturnal enuresis.
5. *Nocturia.* The person is awakened by a need to urinate. This may occur one to five times a night.
6. *Urinary tract infections or cystitis.* Anyone may develop a urinary tract infection. However, when the diagnosis of MS is known, neurogenic bladder should be suspected as the possible cause. Clues to the presence of urinary tract infection include burning or pain during urination (dysuria), increased frequency, urgency, incontinence, foul-smelling urine, pain in the lower back or abdomen, chills, and fever.

The presence of one or more of the preceding symptoms suggests neurogenic bladder but does not indicate the specific abnormality. This must be determined before treatment can begin, as dissimilar impairments can cause the same symptoms and require very different management. In general, bladder dysfunction in MS occurs when (a) the bladder contracts poorly or excessively, (b) the urinary sphincter fails to relax, or (c) the actions of the muscle of the bladder wall and the sphincter are not properly coordinated.

These impairments of bladder function may differ, although the symptoms may be the same. Urgency, frequency, nocturia, and incontinence may be present in various kinds of bladder dysfunction. For this reason, it is crucial to identify the underlying defect. Without knowing the nature of the impairment, some measures to treat the symptoms may seem to be temporarily successful but may actually worsen the bladder's condition.

The three basic kinds of MS neurogenic bladder are storage dysfunction, emptying dysfunction, and combined dysfunction.

Storage Dysfunction

The primary bladder muscle is overactive and signals an urge to urinate when less than 200 ml (less than a cup) of urine has collected in the bladder. This causes urgency, frequency, nocturia, and possibly incontinence.

Emptying Dysfunction

The primary bladder muscle may be weakened and not able to exert enough force to expel all urine from the bladder; the sphincter may be "tight" and hence not able to relax sufficiently to permit complete emptying (the urine left behind is called "residual urine").

The failure-to-store bladder (storage dysfunction) does not allow the normal volume of urine to accumulate and is also referred to as a "small-capacity bladder." Accumulation of a small amount of urine creates the same need to urinate as that experienced by a person with normal bladder function when three to five times that quantity of urine has collected.

The failure-to-empty bladder (emptying dysfunction) may behave in a similar manner, with small amounts of urine being eliminated frequently. However, the retained urine (often not perceived by the individual) may continue to stretch the bladder. The result may be a "large-capacity bladder," which stretches the bladder muscle beyond recovery. At this point symptoms may actually diminish, as the damaged muscle ceases to signal the urge to void when the bladder is full. Urine may back up to the kidneys and cause substantial damage before the disorder is detected. Too often, awareness emerges when kidney involvement has created a crisis situation.

Combined Dysfunction

Some people with MS may present with a "mixed"-type bladder with some elements of both storage and emptying syndromes. (A syndrome is a collection of symptoms and physical findings that fit within a known diagnostic classification.) These cases are also manageable, although a longer trial-and-error period may be needed to determine the most effective management.

DIAGNOSIS OF BLADDER DYSFUNCTION

In order to evaluate the individual situation, the following steps are suggested: (a) detailed history of past and current bladder symptoms; (b) laboratory tests of the urine to detect infection, if present; (c) measurement of the amount of urine voided and the amount left behind (residual urine) after a concentrated effort to urinate voluntarily; and (d) laboratory testing to evaluate directly the ability of the bladder muscle to contract and the sphincter to relax.

Management is guided by these measures. Before the most effective treatment can be determined, a period of adjusting medications and techniques may be required.

Other tests are needed periodically to evaluate the MS patient's bladder function and the condition of his/her urinary tract. Understanding the purposes, procedures, and expected outcomes of these tests should allay fear and encourage the patient to participate actively in the sometimes lengthy process of bladder management.

History

The history of past and current bladder symptoms involves a dialogue between the patient and clinician about urinary problems that have occurred in the past, and the urinary disturbances that are present at the time of the evaluation. These might include the presence of urgency, frequency, nocturia, incontinence, infection, or other symptoms as well as the type of diagnostic studies and procedures done in the past (such as prostate surgery). Former management measures, as well as bowel and sexual function, are discussed. This information will help to determine the best means for treating current problems by understanding the progression of urinary symptoms and the outcome of previous treatments.

Urinalysis

It is important to determine whether infection or a non-MS problem is underlying urinary symptoms. Testing of the urine should be done when infection (UTI) or a problem not related to MS is suspected.

The urine is tested to detect such abnormalities as the presence of bacteria, blood, or sugar. Results can be available within a few hours, and so the test is useful for screening purposes. If this "urinalysis" reveals abnormalities, more specific testing is needed. For example, the findings of many bacteria and white blood cells and a trace of blood suggest a urinary tract infection. However, the particular bacteria that are present and the drug that is most effective against them must be determined. This testing is called a urine culture (to grow the bacteria) and sensitivity tests (to determine the appropriate antibiotic to be used).

Urinary Culture and Sensitivity

A sterile urine specimen is required for culturing. It may be obtained by catheterization or by the "clean-catch" technique, which involves (a) cleansing around the urinary opening, (b) passing a few drops of urine into the toilet to clear the urinary passage, (c) passing urine into a sterile container, and (d) keeping the specimen cold until delivered to the laboratory.

The urine is then placed on a culture medium in the laboratory and set aside for 48 hours to observe the absence or presence of bacterial growth. Should significant growth occur, the bacteria are identified and then tested against a series of antibiotics to determine which is most effective. The end result is identification of the antibiotic(s) that can destroy that organism. When distressing symptoms accompany the infection, a broad-spectrum antibacterial agent may be given to the patient as soon as a urine culture is obtained. When the laboratory report is available several days later, the antibacterial agent may be continued if tests show it to be an effective one or changed if it has not been shown to kill the bacteria that were present.

Residual Urine

Residual urine determination gives the doctor important information about the present state of the patient's urinary system and his/her susceptibility to potentially serious complications. The "flushing" action of urine passing out of the body serves to expel waste, bacteria, and mineral deposits. Accumulated bacteria can multiply and lead to urinary tract infection, and retained mineral deposits may form urinary stones. The more urine left in the bladder after voiding, the greater is the risk of these complications.

Diagnostic Catheterization

The simplest way of determining residual urine is as follows:

1. When a strong desire to urinate is present, the patient attempts to empty the bladder by urinating into a calabrated container such as a measuring cup so that the voided amount may be measured.
2. After urinating, the nurse or physician inserts a thin, hollow tube (catheter) through the urinary opening into the bladder to drain the remaining urine. This procedure is quick, painless, and safe.

It is helpful to know the amount voided as well as the amount of residual urine, as the total amount reflects the bladder capacity, the amount of urine the bladder stores before it signals an urge to void. The combination of the voided volume plus the residual volume provides useful information that contributes to treatment decisions.

This test is utilized periodically to help determine how effective the treatment is. If the amount of residual urine decreases over a period of weeks or months, it indicates improved bladder function. Patients who are catheterizing themselves can provide this information to the physician or nurse, thereby actively participating in the management process.

Radioisotope Renal/Residual Urine Study

Radioisotope renal/residual urine study (RRU) is a safe and accurate method of measuring residual urine and urine flow in addition to providing information about kidney and bladder function. This procedure is a good diagnostic tool for most patients with suspected neurogenic bladder. However, since kidney and bladder stones are not visualized, this test is not useful when stones are suspected. Also, results can be effectively utilized only when a quantitative measurement is done. Unless the exact amount is calculated, the test is not helpful.

Before making an appointment for an RRU (usually with the Nuclear Medicine Dept.), ask whether "estimates" of residual urine are determined (small, moderate, or large amounts) or actual volumes are measured. It may be advantageous to select another facility if only estimates are provided.

No specific preparation for this test is necessary. The patient is well hydrated, and a radioisotope substance is injected intravenously. The patient's bladder is immediately scanned. After approximately 40 minutes of imaging, the patient voids (urinates) and then returns to the table for additional scanning so that residual urine may be calculated.

This procedure lasts about 2 hours and is neither painful nor uncomfortable, although a venous injection is required.

Serial Ultrasound

Ultrasound is also utilized to detect residual urine. Standard ultrasound testing, however, provides only gross estimates of urine volume. Serial ultrasound can safely and precisely measure bladder capacity and residual volume by computing from serial parallel sections of the bladder. As with the radioisotope study, be sure that quantitative results (actual numbers) will be available. Results are of limited value when only broad estimates are provided.

Intravenous Pyelogram/Urogram

The entire urinary tract is visualized when an intravenous pyelogram or urogram, also called an IVP or an IVU, is undergone. This is a radiologic (X-ray) procedure. A special substance is injected into an arm vein; the material then circulates through the body and temporarily settles in the kidneys before it leaves the body in the urine. This allows the entire urinary system to be visualized via X-ray. "Intravenous" refers to injections into a vein; "pyelogram" is a kidney X-ray; and "urogram" describes the X-ray of the urinary system. Therefore IVU more accurately describes the test, although IVP is a better-known term. Both terms refer to the same procedure.

A "postvoiding" study should also be performed, so that residual volume can be determined. This test clearly visualizes the kidneys and can identify stones. It is indicated when complications of the urinary tract are suspected. For a routine screening, previously mentioned tests are preferred, since the IVP/IVU requires laxatives and enemas to empty the bowel so that the urinary system will be clearly visible.

Urodynamic Studies

Urodynamic studies (UDS) determine the pressure, or expulsive force, within the bladder and the capability of the external sphincter to contract or relax at appropriate times. This test is more complicated and expensive than those previously mentioned and is indicated only under the following conditions:

1. There is a history of serious urinary problems, e.g., bladder surgery.
2. Non-MS bladder problems such as those related to diabetes.
3. Determination of bladder capacity and residual urine by tests previously mentioned have not resulted in successful management of symptoms.

Although UDS are infrequently needed, it is reasonable to describe the test for those who may require it. Several techniques are utilized. The specific procedure is primarily determined by institutional protocol, and all variations known to the authors provide useful information.

The patient may be asked to drink a large amount of fluid prior to the test, depending on the technique used. The rectum should be empty, so laxatives or enemas may be advised for individuals prone to constipation. At the time of testing, a catheter is inserted through the urinary opening and left in place. A plug containing electrodes may be inserted into the rectum, or a tiny needle with electrodes may be inserted directly into the urinary sphincter. Following this preparation, the patient rests comfortably while the bladder fills. He then may be called on to attempt bladder emptying, to cough, or to report changes in bladder sensation. The test is safe and painless and is essential in some situations in order to define what is wrong with the various mechanisms involved in voiding.

Cystoscopy

Cystoscopy is useful only when an obstruction other than a tight sphincter is suspected (such as an enlarged prostate in older men) or another non-MS problem such as a polyp or generalized inflammation is suspected. A thin tube with a light and magnifier is passed through the urinary opening so that the inside of the bladder can be examined visually.

BLADDER MANAGEMENT

Storage Dysfunction

The bladder fails to store urine when there is nervous system damage causing contractions of the bladder muscle that result in emptying before the bladder is filled to a normal capacity. The urge to urinate is then experienced when only a small amount of urine is present. The bladder is considered "hyperactive" and to have a small capacity, as urine does not accumulate to the normal volume. The goal of management is to permit bladder filling to occur up to an adequate capacity before the urge to urinate is signaled.

This is accomplished by certain drugs having "anticholinergic" effects. These drugs cause relaxation of the bladder and other smooth muscles (e.g., gallbladder). Some examples are Pro-Banthine, Ditropan, Bentyl, and Tofranil. The specific drug must be prescribed by a physician. Side effects of these drugs are the result of simultaneous slowing down of nervous system activity in other areas, notably the intestine and salivary glands. Therefore, constipation and dry mouth are likely occurrences. Constipation may be managed by measures described later in this chapter in the section dealing with bowel management. Dry mouth may be relieved by sucking on hard candy or using commercial products such as Moi-Stir or Salivart. Blurred vision is an infrequent side effect that should be reported to the physician if it occurs. Most of these medications are administered cautiously to individuals with glaucoma, so the physician should be informed if glaucoma has been diagnosed or is suspected.

Emptying Dysfunction

The failure-to-empty type of bladder dysfunction shows up as an inability to empty the bladder completely during voiding. This may be caused by bladder contractions of insufficient strength or duration to expel all of the urine in the bladder. The most common cause is incoordination of the bladder muscle and the sphincter. This means that when the bladder muscle provides an expulsive force to evacuate urine, the sphincter tightens instead of relaxing, thereby interfering with urination. In this situation the sphincter is referred to as "spastic," or "hyperactive."

Weak bladder muscle contractions in non-MS conditions may be strengthened by drugs such as Urecholine. However, this is not indicated in MS, as beneficial effects are generally short-lived and serious adverse effects can occur. Moreover, a weakened bladder muscle is usually seen together with a hyperactive sphincter. When these drugs are administered to a person with a hyperactive or spastic sphincter, the bladder contracts more forcefully but against a closed sphincter. This damages the bladder muscle and forms "pockets" where urine may collect. This situation predisposes to urinary tract infection. Another danger is that urine can be forced to back up into the kidneys, thereby posing a serious threat to the patient's health.

In mild instances of failure to empty, an antispasticity drug (such as baclofen) may be effective in relaxing the sphincter, thereby helping to release the urine in the bladder. (See Chapter 6 for more detailed information about the various medications used for bladder management.)

Bladder Training

Some affected individuals can train themselves to simulate normal voiding, keeping the following points in mind. Complete voiding is best performed on a toilet seat, as in this position pressure of internal organs does not cause pressure on the urethra and obstruct the outflow of urine. When the bladder is full and the desire to void is present, urine may flow. The flow may not last long enough, and sometimes it may not occur. In that case, the bladder may be stimulated to contract by tapping the lower abdomen. If some urine comes out, the maneuver can be repeated as many times as is necessary until it produces no flow. Gently touching the urinary opening with a piece of toilet tissue may also release some urine. However, in most patients with the failure-to-empty disorder, intermittent catheterization is called for.

Intermittent Catheterization

Intermittent catheterization (IC) is a safe, easy, and effective means of emptying urine from the bladder. It is performed by inserting a thin hollow tube (catheter) through the urinary opening for the purpose of eliminating all of the urine that has collected in the bladder. This is done several times a day to simulate normal voiding.

The primary goals of IC are:

1. To maintain the health of the urinary system. This is accomplished by preventing recurrent urinary tract infections and secondary kidney (renal) impairment by: (a) *Eliminating residual urine.* The inability to empty the bladder completely at each voiding provides a favorable medium for bacterial growth—similar to a stagnant pool of water—thereby fostering the development of urinary tract infections. Continuous or recurrent bladder infections may eventually involve the kidneys and create a serious health problem. (b) *Preventing bladder distention.* Filling the bladder beyond normal capacity reduces the bladder's inherent ability to fight off infection. The bladder muscle stretches, similar to a balloon that is filled with so much air that its walls become very thin. When this occurs with the bladder, its muscle fibers are stretched beyond their ability to function. Thus, the weakened muscle cannot effectively expel urine, and large amounts of stagnant urine are retained. This process may be reversible if muscle fibers have not been destroyed by too much stretching. The sooner the process of bladder stretching is reversed, the more likely it is that recovery can occur. (c) *Preventing kidney damage caused by reflux.* Urine in a distended bladder may be forced back up

the ureters toward the kidneys (reflux). Infected urine makes this particularly dangerous, as a kidney infection may result.
2. Improve patient function. Periodic complete emptying of the bladder often relieves complaints of urgency, frequency, nocturia, and incontinence, especially when combined with appropriate medication. The length of time between urinating should be increased, and "accidents" may be eliminated.
3. Restore bladder function. Periodic emptying of the distended bladder frequently promotes the return of bladder muscle strength. Following 3 to 4 months of IC, bladder function may approach normal, eliminating the need for continuing IC. Although restoration of function is not possible for everyone, it is considered a goal during the evaluation and management process.

Technique

Although IC is generally considered valuable, various techniques are used. Most health professionals who teach IC to patients in the community advise some form of the "clean" technique. This means that strict sterile practices (such as the use of sterile gloves) are not required. The rationale is that the bladder has a natural tendency to resist infection so long as it is emptied periodically, and any bacteria introduced with the catheter are flushed out with the urine. The basic guidelines for the patient performing IC are as follows:

1. Wash the hands.
2. Attempt to urinate.
3. Clean around the urinary opening with soap and water.
4. Insert a lubricated catheter (#14 French for women, #12 French for men) and drain the urine.
5. Remove the catheter and either discard or wash and store it.
6. Periodically measure the amount urinated and the residual urine, keeping a dated record of these numbers. Voided and residual amounts provide an ongoing assessment of bladder function and will help the physician or nurse determine when IC can be decreased or discontinued.

For those patients who require IC several times a day, the technique should be designed to fit comfortably into the daily routine. When IC is performed on a regular basis, relief of symptoms encourages continuation of the procedure. For men, the urinary opening is visible, and the technique is easily mastered by those with the ability to use their hands. Women, however, have the urethral opening (meatus) located outside of direct vision. This situation is approached in the same manner as learning to insert a tampon. A mirror should be used to identify the meatus. During practice sessions, inserting a tampon into the vagina is helpful; with the vagina blocked, only one opening is left for inserting the catheter (Fig. 2). Continued use of a mirror needlessly complicates the technique.

Both men and women may meet resistance when attempting to insert the catheter. This results from a spastic or tight sphincter, which will usually relax if the person pauses a few seconds, attempts to relax, and then continues. Passing a catheter may also produce transient spasms of the legs. Should this occur, pause for a few seconds until the leg spasms pass and continue catheter insertion. Clear plastic or rubber catheters may be used. For those individuals who have problems with their hands, the plastic catheters are more rigid and easier to insert.

Intermittent catheterization may need to be performed by someone other than the patient when severe motor or sensory disability interferes with self-insertion. A family member or home attendant may be taught to perform this function. Intermittent catheterization is far preferable to a catheter that is left in the bladder, as the latter has the greater risk of complications.

Additional applications of IC should be noted. Women who experience incontinence during sexual intercourse can perform IC prior to sexual activity. Also, those who utilize IC on a regular basis may alter their schedule when desired (such as prior to a shopping expedition). This flexibility enhances the person's control over his/her bladder function. The physician will often prescribe a urinary antiseptic such as Mandelamine or Hiprex to aid in the prevention of urinary tract infection. These drugs help to acidify the urine, which deters growth of most bacteria that cause urinary infections. Vitamin C, 1,000 mg

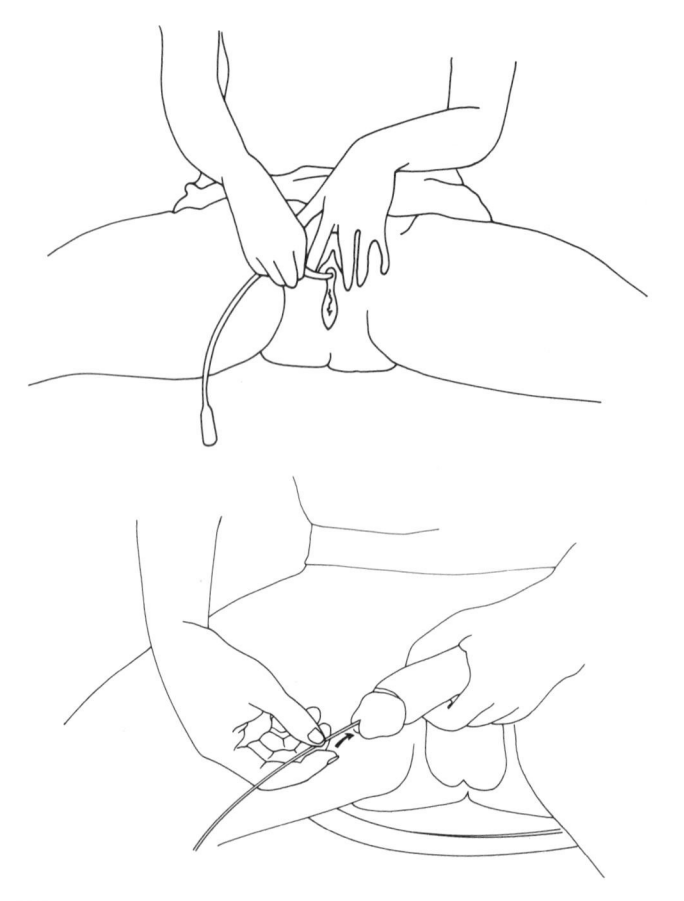

FIG. 2. Female **(top)** and male **(bottom)** self-catheterization.

four times per day, also helps acidify the urine, as do cranberry juice and prune juice. Citrus juices (orange, grapefruit, and tomato) should be limited, since they promote alkaline urine despite their vitamin C content.

Combined Bladder Dysfunction

The combined neurogenic bladder has features of both the failure-to-store and failure-to-empty disorders. The sphincter is tight and does not allow the bladder to empty completely. However, even when the

BLADDER AND BOWEL MANAGEMENT

patient can empty his/her bladder (usually because IC is done), the hyperactive bladder signals the urge to urinate when only a small amount of urine has collected. Medication is needed to relax the bladder and allow a normal amount of urine to collect. The bladder can then be emptied by conveniently scheduled IC.

It is important to realize that bladder symptoms fluctuate. They are usually not progressive and often improve over periods of time, especially when proper treatment is initiated early.

INDWELLING CATHETERS

There are certain situations when it is best to use a catheter that remains inside the bladder. The usual type of this "indwelling catheter" is called a "Foley catheter." This is a thin, hollow tube that is inserted into the bladder and connected to an external drainage bag. The catheter is kept in the bladder by a small balloon that is inflated after insertion. The catheter is easily removed by deflating this balloon through an external valve.

The conditions that might indicate a need for temporary use of an indwelling catheter are as follows:

1. A person whose bladder has been excessively stretched by urinary retention for several months may benefit from a few weeks of this type of urinary drainage. Although IC is preferred, it is not always possible because of the person's severe disability and the absence of someone else to carry out the procedure on a regular basis. The expectation is that the bladder muscle may regain some degree of normal function by relieving the pressure and stretching caused by urinary retention.
2. When someone other than the MS person performs IC, and it is necessary for this individual to be absent for several days or more, a Foley catheter may have to be used.
3. If pressure sores develop on the buttocks or other areas close to the urinary opening, a Foley catheter may be needed to eliminate urinary incontinence, a factor that impedes healing of the pressure sores.
4. Following surgical procedures that involve the urinary or reproductive systems or after difficult childbirth, indwelling catheteriza-

tion may be needed until the swelling of surrounding tissues subsides and urinary flow may resume unobstructed.
5. Certain social or travel situations may present obstacles to urination or to IC. Important social functions (such as weddings) may not be held in places with accessible toilets. This is also usually true with various travel modes as well (bus, train, airplane). A Foley catheter may be a comfortable way of overcoming such barriers to pleasurable experiences. Ideally, a catheter in these situations should not be left in for more than 24 hours. Beyond this time, bacterial growth in the bladder is almost inevitable and increases the risk of bladder infection.

Some of the situations that necessitate long-term indwelling catheterization include the following:

1. Severe disability that precludes self-catheterization or the unavailability of another individual who can perform IC on a regular basis.
2. Female incontinence resistant to any other type of control.
3. Women who are at great risk from their susceptibility to skin ulceration and need to avoid any possibility of urinary incontinence.
4. Obese women who are unable to stand and cannot transfer, alone or assisted, to a toilet or commode because of excessive body weight.
5. Females who are prevented by emotional or intellectual disturbances from participating in alternative measures of bladder management.

Indwelling catheterization is prescribed more often for women than men. This is because of sex-related anatomical differences rather than "sex discrimination." The penis provides a convenient appendage for attachment of an external drainage device. This is not as effective for females because of the location of their urinary opening.

Care of Indwelling Catheters

The indwelling catheter can be managed at home with minimal effort. It is inserted using sterile technique and is changed every 4 to 6 weeks or more frequently if blockage occurs. The community's visiting nurse association will generally provide this service when it is requested by a physician. The catheter insertion kit should be obtained prior to the nurse's visit. Other supplies needed are a leg bag, a night bag, a washcloth, mild soap, alcohol, an irrigation set, saline solution, and vinegar.

Daily care consists of cleaning around the catheter insertion site with soap and water in the morning and the evening. An individual with an indwelling catheter needs to drink an adequate or even an excessive amount of fluids—2 to 3 quarts a day. Fluids should be selected that promote urinary acidity, thereby deterring bacterial growth. This excludes such juices as orange, grapefruit, and tomato while encouraging intake of cranberry, apple, apricot, and prune juices. Vitamin C, at a dose of 1,000 mg four times a day, is also recommended for this purpose. A urinary antiseptic is also advised but must be prescribed by a physician.

When changing from the leg bag worn during the day to a night bag, connecting pieces should be wiped with alcohol to impede the entrance of bacteria. Collection bags (leg and night) can be rinsed with warm water and then deodorized by a mixture of warm water and vinegar left soaking in the bag for a few hours.

Leakage of urine around the catheter tube or expulsion of the catheter has several possible causes, and these must be systematically examined:

1. *Obstructed catheter drainage.* The small drainage holes of the catheter may become blocked by mucus or sediment, requiring irrigation to clear the passageway. The irrigation set and saline are utilized for this purpose. The procedure can be carried out by the visiting nurse or by an individual in the household instructed in the proper technique.
2. *Adequate fluid intake.* If insufficient fluid is drunk, the urine will be concentrated and may serve as an irritant to the bladder, causing vigorous contractions, which force urine out around the drainage tube. It is essential that fluid intake be at least 2 to 3 quarts a day.
3. *Urinary tract infection.* Infected urine may act as an irritant, stimulating bladder contractions. If this occurs, a urine specimen must be checked in the laboratory for the presence of bacteria: a culture and sensitivity test should be done.

4. *Bladder muscle spasms.* The neurogenic bladder may have uninhibited spasms that intermittently force urine out around the catheter. This may be controlled by medication such as Pro-Banthine or Ditropan.
5. *Oversized catheter or retaining balloon.* A catheter or retaining balloon that is too large is irritating and causes inflammation, which may lead to infection. An oversized catheter or balloon is sometimes unfortunately used as a "plug" to control leakage without exploring possible causes. Other long-term problems may result when an oversized catheter is used inappropriately.
6. *Bladder stones.* Indwelling catheters increase the risk of stone formation and subsequent bladder irritation leading to leakage. A cystoscopy (direct visualization of the inside of the bladder) is used to detect and remove bladder stones.

SURGICAL PROCEDURES

There are no surgical procedures that can return the bladder to normal functioning. The primary goals of therapy are to promote bladder emptying, relieve symptoms, and subsequently reduce debilitating, possibly life-threatening complications. A few surgical procedures can help achieve these goals under special circumstances. The most common are suprapubic cystostomy, sphincterotomy, and transurethral resection.

Cystostomy

Cystostomy is a surgically created opening into the urinary bladder through the lower abdomen. A catheter is inserted through the new opening and connected by plastic tubing to a collection device (leg bag/night bag). Urine flows through the catheter rather than through the natural urinary opening. The operation is not a major procedure and requires the patient to be in a hospital for only a few days.

The reasons for using this approach are similar to those calling for the use of a permanent indwelling catheter. Moreover, it is easily taken care of—in a fashion similar to that for the urethral catheter—and injuries to the urethra may be avoided. Cystostomy is only occasionally necessary. An additional measure is use of a gauze pad cut to surround the cystostomy tube and held in place with hypoallergenic tape.

Sphincterotomy

In the severely spastic male who cannot empty his bladder despite all efforts, the sphincter can be enlarged surgically. An inability to control urination results, but it can be managed in males by an external collecting device. Females are not candidates for the procedure because urinary drainage cannot be managed without the danger of skin breakdown.

Transurethral Resection

When a patient has had an indwelling catheter for a long time and the pressure of the balloon of the Foley catheter has irritated the bladder neck (the area where the bladder connects with the urethra), the tissues may become thickened and obstruct the flow of urine when the catheter is removed. In that case, the excess tissue of the bladder neck is removed, which then allows the urine to flow freely. The procedure is required only rarely and most often in males.

There are other procedures that may be advocated, but most of them are indicated only rarely and should be undertaken with careful consideration.

PRODUCTS FOR MANAGING URINARY INCONTINENCE

Although urinary incontinence can be eliminated for most persons with MS, some do continue to have loss of control over urination despite all medical efforts. Also, for the person who has achieved urinary control, special circumstances (e.g., urinary tract infection, inaccessible bathrooms) may result in temporary incontinence. The following products are useful in minimizing the embarrassing and potentially harmful effects (e.g., skin ulceration) of incontinence.

Male External Catheters

The most popular external male catheter is the condom catheter, which is similar in design to the condom utilized for birth control. Several sizes and styles are available, e.g., Texas catheter, Urosan, Freedom catheter. Some external catheters are designed for one-time use, and others are reusable. For long-term use, a reusable and inexpensive external catheter can be made from a condom and a section of rubber tubing. Instructions for making this device can be obtained by contacting the authors. Care must be taken to ensure that strips holding the catheter in place are applied loosely enough to allow full blood circulation and not irritate the skin (Fig. 3).

The Mentor Hold-Free Glans Cap is designed to fit on the head of the penis (glans). This may be useful as a temporary measure if there is irritation on the shaft of the penis. The best method is for the person to try several different brands and choose the one best suited for him.

Male "drip collectors" are designed to absorb small amounts of urine (up to 3 oz). Conveen, for the male, is a disposable, absorbent "pocket" that fits around the penis.

Female Collection Devices

Female external urinary collection (Misstique), a specially contoured silicone device, is designed to fit snugly around the urinary opening and is held in place by a silicone sealant. A panty and liner provide additional security and comfort. The device is attached to a connective tubing and drainage bag. This is a new device that shows promise for controlling female urinary incontinence but has not been marketed long enough for potential problems to be identified.

Drainage Bags

The external device is attached to a connecting tube and drainage bag. Leg drainage bags come in varying sizes and are secured to the calf of the leg by straps. The smaller size is more easily concealed.

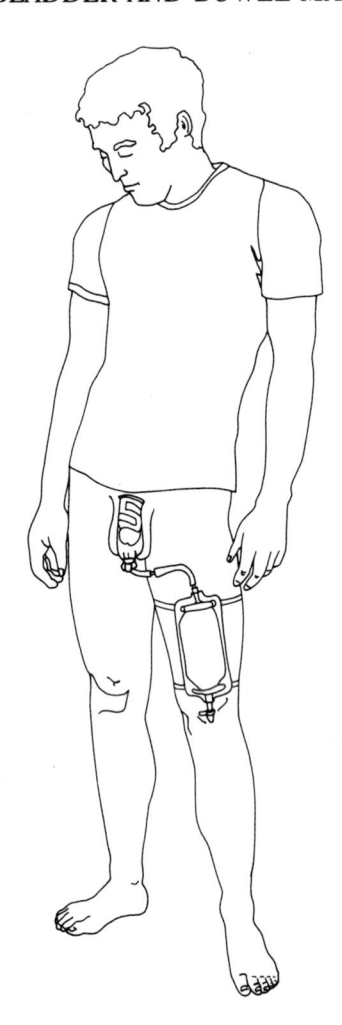

FIG. 3. Condom catheter.

However, it requires more frequent emptying than the larger bag. The "sport" bag is worn horizontally across the thigh rather than vertically along the calf and permits the wearing of shorts or skirts. The sport bag is better for use by ambulatory persons, as a seated person is not in a good position to allow for gravity drainage. Leg bags should not be worn by a person who is confined to bed.

"Night" bags are available, which are attached to the bed, promoting drainage by their position below the level of the bladder. Drainage bag guidelines also apply to indwelling catheters such as Foleys or cystostomy tubes.

Diapers and Briefs

Designed for one-time use only, these highly absorbent diaper-type products are available in various styles and sizes, e.g., Attends, Tranquility, Depends.

Lightweight reusable pants are available with disposable highly absorbent pads, which slip into the panty or briefs, e.g., Dignity, Kanga, Confidence.

Unproven therapies, which have not been shown to be of value in multiple sclerosis and have surgical risks, include bladder pacemaker, dorsal column stimulator, artificial sphincter, and continent vesicostomy.

Biofeedback is being studied as a possible aid to control urinary incontinence. It is not known at this time whether it will be shown to be an effective procedure.

BOWEL MANAGEMENT

Most people with MS gave little thought to bowel function before the onset of their illness. Many continue without bowel dysfunction throughout the course of the disease. However, for those who are currently having bowel problems, or who have an interest in understanding the causes and management of bowel dysfunction in MS, this section is relevant.

The most common bowel complaint of the person with MS is constipation. There are several factors that cause or contribute to this problem. However, regardless of the underlying cause or causes, management measures are the same. Loss of bowel control (bowel incontinence) is an infrequent but very disturbing occurrence in MS.

Constipation

Constipation is defined as a condition in which bowel movements are infrequent or incomplete. "Infrequent" bowel movement is defined as occurring less often than every 3 days. "Incomplete" refers to part or most of the stool being retained in the rectum or lower intestine following attempts to have a bowel movement (defecate). Perception as to what is normal needs to be examined in light of this. It is not necessary to have a daily bowel movement, but defecation once a week or less often is outside the acceptable range. Stool that is increasingly retained in the lower digestive tract tends to stretch the bowel, thereby weakening its ability to move waste out of the body. Also, the longer the stool is retained in the intestine, the more of its water content is withdrawn by the body. This creates a dry, hardened stool, which is increasingly difficult to evacuate.

In addition to the obvious effects of constipation, more subtle events also occur. Stool retained in the rectum may cause pressure on parts of the urinary system, thereby increasing bladder disturbance. Stretching of the rectum by retained stool sends messages to the spinal cord, which further disturbs bladder function and adversely affects walking because of increased spasticity. This information is important, as many people view constipation as a localized annoyance. Understanding this pattern enhances awareness of the benefits of an effective bowel program for individuals with MS.

Constipation may result directly from MS involvement of that portion of the nervous system that controls bowel function. This produces a "sluggish bowel," which moves waste slowly through the digestive system. As with incomplete emptying, the body then absorbs a greater amount of water from the stool (feces), leaving hardened stool, which is difficult to pass. Another indirect MS influence on bowel movements is weakened abdominal muscles. This makes it difficult to "bear down" strongly enough to create sufficient pressure within the abdomen for easy evacuation of stool. The result is constipation.

Decreased physical activity because of impaired walking or easy fatigability is a common secondary cause of sluggish bowel activity. Constipation also results when the amount of fluid a person drinks is voluntarily reduced. This most often happens when urinary complaints, such as urgency, frequency, and loss of control (incontinence), are present. In this situation, fluid restriction is intended to minimize urinary problems, although constipation is a predictable outcome. Another contributing factor is postponement of defecation once awareness of a full rectum is experienced. Certain types of drugs are also known to promote constipation. These include pain relievers containing narcotics (such as codeine) and some medications used to treat urinary symptoms.

Chronic harsh laxative use eventually increases constipation. As the laxative effect wears off, there is a "rebound" reaction of the bowel to a more sluggish state than prior to the laxative use.

Management is discussed here by first outlining general measures to promote good bowel function. This is followed by specific measures, listed according to the order in which they should be utilized. An adequate trial should be attempted at each level. An important point is that any trial of bowel management requires several weeks before effectiveness can be evaluated, as a gradual modification of the digestive rhythm is involved.

General Measures to Promote Good Bowel Function

1. Adequate fluid intake of at least 2 quarts a day. Include coffee, juice, or whatever fluids are desired.
2. Daily intake of fiber (such as unprocessed bran) to provide water-retaining bulk in the stool. This stimulates movement of the stool toward the rectum.
3. Regular physical activity including exercise. This may range from swimming to wheelchair exercises. Whatever physical activity is reasonable for the individual will be helpful.
4. Evacuation at the same time of day. The best time to attempt defecation is one-half hour after mealtime, when the emptying reflex (gastrocolic reflex) is strongest.

Measures to Manage Resistant Constipation

1. All of the above.
2. Stool softeners (such as Colace) daily.

BLADDER AND BOWEL MANAGEMENT

3. Bulk supplements (natural fiber supplements) such as Metamucil daily.
4. Mild oral laxatives, such as milk of magnesia, on alternate nights or nightly if needed.
5. Glycerin suppository one-half hour prior to planned evacuation. This may be needed for several weeks during the period of regulating the bowel, or it may be used indefinitely.
6. Bisocodyl (Dulcolax) suppositories when glycerin suppositories have proved ineffective.
7. Fleet enema at the time of planned evacuation periodically when usual measures have been ineffective or on a regular basis if absolutely necessary. This measure is used in conjunction with stool softeners, bulk supplements, and mild oral laxatives.

Measures to Manage Severe and Long-Standing Constipation in the Severely Disabled Person

1. An adequate trial of all the above measures.
2. Medical evaluation to check out possible contributing factors other than MS.
3. Tap water enema every 2 to 3 days in conjunction with previously mentioned fluid intake, dietary fiber, stool softeners, laxatives, and/or suppositories as indicated by the benefit observed. The tap water enema may also be used periodically when routinely practiced measures are ineffective.
4. Manual removal of hardened feces in the rectum by inserting the index and middle fingers into the rectum (rubber glove and lubricant required). This is an infrequently needed technique for the severely debilitated person who is normally regulated by other measures.

An additional technique for individuals who find it difficult to completely empty the rectum is digital stimulation of the anal opening. Insertion of the index finger (covered with a latex "finger cot") through the anal sphincter, with gentle rotation of the finger, may be sufficient to stimulate rectal emptying. The technique should be used only periodically, as chronic anal stretching may cause damage to the anal sphincter. It is also important to note the impact of varying dietary habits on bowel function. Individuals differ in their response to specific foods, and this needs to be considered when determining an overall bowel program.

Bowel Incontinence

Total loss of bowel control is a rare occurrence in MS, but it does affect some severely disabled individuals. Episodic loss of bowel control, however, can occur when there is only minimal MS impairment. This is a very distressing and difficult problem to resolve.

Bowel incontinence occurs (a) when there is loose stool and intestinal upset, such as when the patient has flu; (b) when MS affects the intestine or anal sphincter; and (c) occasionally when non-MS-related bowel problems are present. Therefore, when a fair trial of regulatory measures is unsuccessful or when bowel incontinence persists beyond an acute flu-type illness, a gastroenterologist (a doctor specializing in gastrointestinal disorders) should be consulted. Non-MS bowel problems may be then identified and treated with a greater degree of success.

Loose stool present during episodes of incontinence may be responsible for the bowel accidents, as the anal sphincter cannot easily contain liquid. Loose stool may result from common viral or flu-type syndromes, and in those instances the problem will solve itself. Dietary factors may be the cause for some individuals, and a test elimination of substances that irritate the gut (such as spicy food, coffee, alcohol, and cigarettes) may be effective. Loose stool can also be passed around a blockage of hardened feces in the lower intestine or rectum. This blockage is called impaction and requires aggressive efforts, including an oil retention enema or tap water enema, for correction. Establishment of an effective bowel program that is followed faithfully usually prevents recurrence of this problem.

Multiple sclerosis involvement that is responsible for occasional, or in some severely disabled persons frequent, loss of bowel control can be caused by sensory loss in the rectum. Rectal filling may be partially or totally unperceived, allowing the rectum to stretch beyond the usual capacity. An unexpected, involuntary relaxation of the anal sphincter may occur, resulting in bowel incontinence. The most effective way (currently known) to combat this problem is to establish a regular bowel program and stay with it. When the bowel is trained to empty at regular intervals, accidents are less likely.

In these cases the measures for bowel regulation will include those used to manage constipation. Adequate fluid intake, fiber in the diet, exercise, and possibly a suppository to stimulate a bowel movement at the scheduled time exemplify a possible program. An important point is that a daily bowel movement is not necessary—the regularity of the time interval (such as every other day) and the time of day (such as always after breakfast) are the important time factors.

During the period of bowel training (which may be several weeks or months), while incontinence is a concern, a few suggestions may be helpful. It is very important to be alert to signals that suggest the need to defecate about 30 minutes after meals. A reflex that encourages bowel emptying (gastrocolic reflex) occurs at this time, suggesting that this is a prime time for an accident if one is likely to occur. Also, coffee and other hot liquids may stimulate a rapid response from the digestive system and a precipitous urge to defecate. The physician may prescribe medication (anticholinergic) that relaxes hyperactive bowel and helps to reduce the chance of bowel incontinence.

For these individuals who find bowel incontinence a frequent problem, protective underpants are recommended. An absorbant lining helps protect the skin, and a plastic outer shield inhibits release of odor and shields clothing from being soiled. For persistent incontinence, a drainable fecal incontinence collector (Hollister) may be indicated, especially for those individuals who are confined to bed. The collector is constructed from odor-barrier material and keeps discharge away from the skin.

Some innovative ways to control bowel incontinence are being explored, such as biofeedback. This technique involves sensitizing the individual to subtle signals of rectal filling to compensate for diminished normal mechanisms. Although this technique is still in the exploratory stage, it exemplifies the possibilities for management that may be available in the near future.

Bowel management is often a tedious, frustrating experience. Trial and error is usually involved, and success may be measured by small accomplishments at infrequent intervals. However, persistence is usually rewarded with some sense of control over bowel function and a subsequent release from the continuing worry over the effects of bowel dysfunction.

SUMMARY

Problems with urination and bowel function occur in the majority of individuals with MS at some time during the course of the disease. Symptoms in these areas frequently remit and should not be viewed as a permanent disability. Successful management is possible in most cases. Symptoms can be relieved, complications prevented, and irreversible damage to the urinary tract and bowel avoided. However, the MS person must openly communicate the specific symptoms to the physician and be aggressive in seeking the necessary help.

12

Sexuality

Rosalind C. Kalb, Nicholas G. LaRocca, and Seymour R. Kaplan

Sexuality is an important part of life and of relating to others. It plays a significant role in determining how a person feels about him- or herself. The average person between the ages of 20 and 50 today faces a variety of complex pressures in relation to sex. Most people bring from childhood certain taboos or inhibitions that make it difficult to discuss sexual problems or feelings. At the same time, the current social/sexual milieu in our culture places a heavy emphasis on sexual expression, openness, and experimentation.

This apparent contradiction has both negative and positive implications for the disabled person. On the one hand, an MS patient confronted with a variety of sexual problems may have no one (perhaps not even a spouse) with whom he or she can comfortably talk about sexual matters. The individual may not even be comfortable thinking about these problems. This difficulty is then compounded by the current emphasis on sexuality and freedom of sexual expression. The individual is left feeling inadequate and frustrated, with no place to turn for help. From a more positive perspective, however, the current emphasis on sexual freedom may make it easier for the individual with sexual problems to consider varied or alternative modes of sexual expression.

Sexual intercourse in the more traditional man-on-top position is no longer the only "acceptable" means of expressing one's sexuality. Many individuals, with or without disability, are feeling freer to engage in oral or anal sex, masturbatory activities with or without a partner, or other sexual activities that they find satisfying and pleasurable. The current popular literature is filled with sexual how-to books, which describe varied ways of giving and receiving sexual pleasure and satisfaction before, during, or apart from intercourse.

Multiple sclerosis is a complex and difficult disease that requires an ongoing, open relationship between the person with the disease and his or her sexual partner. The material presented here may serve as a useful tool in this dialogue rather than as a substitute for it. All too frequently, sexual difficulties are ignored or denied because neither partner feels comfortable acknowledging or discussing them.

Sexual problems also need to be discussed with a physician or other knowledgeable and supportive health care professional. Such individuals may prove to be valuable resources in the ongoing coping process. Unfortunately, physicians often ignore sexual problems or hesitate to question their patients about this sensitive issue. The MS person may need to take the initiative in discussing sexual problems with the doctor. The joint efforts of patient, partner, and physician need to be directed toward accomplishing the succcessful and satisfying management of whatever sexual problems may develop.

NORMAL SEXUAL FUNCTIONING

Sexual response occurs in two separate phases, which are similar in both men and women. The first phase involves vasocongestion. In males, blood is carried to, and trapped within, special parts of the penis, causing it to become erect. Similarly in the female, swelling occurs in the blood vessels of the labia and tissues of the vagina, resulting in vaginal lubrication and expansion of the vaginal walls. This initial arousal phase can occur in response to two types of stimulation: physical contact including kissing and caressing, and erotic thoughts or mental images. Arousal in response to mental images is said to be psychogenic in origin and is controlled by the higher brain centers.

Orgasm is the second phase of sexual response. In males, orgasm consists of two phases, emission and ejaculation. Emission is the reflex contraction of the internal reproduction organs, experienced by men as the sensation of imminent ejaculation. Emission is followed almost immediately by ejaculation, a series of contractions of the muscles at the base of the penis. In contrast, the female orgasm involves only one process consisting of a similar series of muscle contractions.

Following orgasm males experience a refractory period of variable length during which sexual arousal is reduced and they are unable to reach another orgasm. Females, however, have no such refractory period. They can usually have repeated orgasms without a reduction in arousal level.

SEXUAL DIFFICULTIES RELATED TO MS

Sexual functioning of persons with MS may be profoundly influenced by the physical and emotional effects of the disease. Lilius surveyed 302 people with MS and found that 91% of the men and 77% of the women reported a change in their sexual lives. Only 20% of the men in their survey reported an adequate erection. Women mentioned inability to achieve orgasm (33%), loss of libido (27%), and spasticity interfering with sex (12%) as their chief difficulties. Clearly, sexual functioning represents an area of concern for people with MS. Although these statistics may appear distressing, two important points should be kept in mind. First, people with MS are not alone in experiencing sexual problems. In any typical "happily married" sample of individuals, a large percentage report sexual problems, many of which are similar to some of the difficulties related to MS. Second, "successful" sex does not have to be defined as having an erection, having intercourse, or having an orgasm. The satisfaction achieved in sexual contact comes from three major sources: pleasurable physical sensations, affectionate closeness with another person, and the gratifying feeling of performing successfully and giving pleasure. The potential problems caused by MS can, of course, interfere with any one or all of these sources of satisfaction at one time or another.

The aim here is to demonstrate how people can learn to achieve satisfaction in varying ways when and if the need arises and perhaps even to redefine for themselves what feels good or is sexually satisfying. The remainder of this chapter points out the difficulties most frequently reported by individuals with MS. The problems fall into four major areas: (a) those resulting from the neurophysiological changes of MS;

(b) those caused by possible physical changes; (c) psychological conflicts and pressures related to disability; and (d) problems resulting from social pressures and attitudes.

Although it is useful for individuals with MS and their sexual partners to understand the various causes of their sexual problems, it may be even more useful and satisfying to learn how others have successfully tackled these problems.

SEXUAL DIFFICULTIES RELATED TO THE NEUROPHYSIOLOGICAL CHANGES OF MS

Because MS may affect many parts of the central nervous system, almost any part of the sexual response may be affected. Multiple sclerosis may impair a person's ability to become sexually aroused, resulting in unsatisfactory penile erection or vaginal lubrication. However, even in those individuals in whom this arousal response is impaired, a reflex response may remain. For example, the person might be unable to achieve erection via sexual thoughts but respond with a reflex erection when the penis is stroked. Other individuals experience the opposite phenomenon. The perineal (genital area) reflex may be lost, but the person can still become sexually aroused in response to visual or emotional stimulation.

Sensations in the genital area may be totally or partially lost because of MS. When the sensations are only partly lost, stimulation that at one time felt good may begin to feel irritating or even painful. These sensory changes can interfere with a person's ability to feel pleasurable sensations, and this in turn can interfere with the ability to ejaculate or have an orgasm. Problems in the autonomic nervous system—the system that controls automatic, nonvoluntary bodily actions (such as digestion)—can also cause problems with erection or vaginal lubrication. If MS has affected the "higher" brain centers—those involved in thoughts and emotions—there may be changes in sexual desire and arousal. Other changes in these same centers may interfere with a person's ability to communicate clearly with the sexual partner.

It is clear from these examples that MS can produce a variety of central nervous system changes that directly affect the sexual response.

Like other MS symptoms caused by changes in the central nervous system, these neurologically based changes in sexual feelings have no absolute "cure." However, it is often possible to circumvent these problems through some combination of creativity, flexibility, and possible sexual aids and/or prosthetic devices.

The neurologically caused erectile and ejaculatory difficulties experienced by many men with MS generally do not remit, although their frequency or regularity of occurrence differs from one individual to another. The first step in the management of these difficulties is a frank discussion with a health professional who is familiar with multiple sclerosis and its symptoms. This individual can help the person with MS determine to what extent the difficulties are a result of neurological impairment and what role psychological factors (such as performance anxiety or depression) may be playing. The man with MS can help in the evaluation effort by becoming familiar with his own body and its functioning. The following are questions he needs to ask himself and be ready to answer for the doctor: "Am I able to achieve and maintain an erection by any means, either during intercourse or through masturbation?" "Do I ever awaken in the night or early morning with an erection?" If the answer to either of these questions is "yes," neurological impairment is probably not total. This means that the person can sometimes achieve and maintain an erection by direct stimulation of the penis. If the answer to the questions is "no," neurological impairment is likely to be more extensive, and the problems may be more permanent. An additional question the person needs to ask himself is: "Am I experiencing bowel or bladder difficulties, such as feelings of urgency, frequency of urination, or incontinence?" In MS, sexual problems caused by neurological changes frequently occur in conjunction with bowel and bladder problems.

The evaluation process used to determine this may involve a detailed interview as well as actual tests of erectile functioning. One such test, which can be performed at home, is the Dacomed Snap-Gauge band. A tape is placed around the penis at night for three or four consecutive days in order to measure the number and rigidity of nocturnal erections. Since the average male has four to five erections nightly, the tape will indicate whether or not such erections occur. If none occur during sleep, it is safe to assume that the problem is neurological in origin rather than emotional. If the band demonstrates that erections occur during sleep, the man can assume that neurological impairment is not total—that the erectile response can still occur. Unfortunately, the presence of nocturnal erections in no way guarantees that penile rigidity will be sufficient for sexual intercourse. In other words, it is possible to have a degree of neurological impairment that results in partial, transitory, or sporadic erections. Under these uncertain circumstances, the neurological and psychological causes of impotence become intertwined, as the man worries each time about his ability to "perform" successfully.

The second step in the management of erectile problems involves specific techniques. In those individuals who can achieve reflex erections by stroking the penis, intercourse is possible, though probably without ejaculation. This can be a satisfying solution for those men who can derive sexual pleasure primarily from pleasing their partners. If a man is able to have an erection or feel physically aroused only infrequently, it will be important for him to learn how to identify those times and take advantage of them. Here again, awareness of his own body and the ability to share this with his partner is necessary.

Men should be aware that orgasm may occur without visible ejaculation. This is caused by retrograde ejaculation, in which the semen is ejaculated back into the bladder. This may be alarming to the person but is not harmful. Retrograde ejaculation does prevent conception, however, and couples who wish to have children should discuss this problem with a urologist or a fertility specialist.

Penile prostheses are a possible alternative for men with chronic erectile problems who strongly wish to engage in intercourse. These protheses are implanted surgically by a urologist. Currently there are three main types of prosthesis, each with its own advantages and disadvantages. The noninflatable rod-type prosthesis consists of two sponge-filled rods that are surgically inserted into the shaft of the penis. These rods create a permanent semierection. The advantages of this prosthesis include a relatively simple and inexpensive surgical procedure that requires less than a week of hospitalization and is associated with few complications. With the rod-type device, however, the penis is constantly semierect and therefore difficult to conceal. Also, the penis is smaller than it is with an inflatable device (see below), and problems can occur that require reimplantation.

A newer type of prosthetic device is a flexible version of the rod-type implant. A flexible silver rod coated with soft plastic is implanted into the penile shaft. The penis remains in a constant semierect state but can be bent upward at the angle of an erect penis or downward at the nonerect angle for easier concealment.

The inflatable-type prosthesis has more advantages and disadvantages than the rod-type implants. The erection process with this device simulates the normal process and therefore allows greater psychological satisfaction. The newest version of the inflatable prosthesis contains its own pressure transducer. This allows the penis to become erect in an apparently "normal" fashion simply by changing its position. The erect penis is larger than it is with the rod device and has a normal nonerect appearance when not inflated. The inpatient implantation procedure takes under an hour. The device does not interfere with urinary function. The inflatable prosthesis, however, is relatively expensive, and the newest model still seems to provide less than optimum penile rigidity. The penile implants do carry with them some risk of infection, which needs to be discussed fully with the physician.

Women who experience difficulties becoming aroused or reaching orgasm because of neurological changes are also encouraged to talk problems over with a knowledgeable health care professional and to become as familiar as possible with their own bodies. If and when sexual feelings and sensations change, each woman can then learn for herself and convey to her partner what is and is not pleasurable to her. Such changes in women, even if temporary, can nevertheless be frustrating and uncomfortable, making open communication with the partner essential.

Women who are experiencing decreased vaginal lubrication should use a sterile, water-soluble jelly such as K-Y. Vaseline should never be used because it is not water-soluble and may cause severe urinary tract infection.

Painful genital sensations in either men or women are best relieved by the same medications used for other sensory problems of MS such as trigeminal neuralgia (facial pain) or assorted paresthesias (sensations of burning, tingling, crawling, or constriction). Tegretol (carbamazepine) is the drug of choice for these problems, with Dilantin (phenytoin) as a second choice when Tegretol is not effective. If disturbing or painful genital sensations have replaced pleasurable ones, or pleasurable sensations are lost because of numbness or anesthesia in the genital area, individuals can learn to identify other areas of their bodies that respond sexually. This process occurs through experimentation and frank discussion with the sexual partner. Individuals and couples who are forced to be innovative often "discover" parts of their bodies and sexual techniques they had never before thought of or tried. Oral and manual stimulation of different parts of the body can often be a very satisfying alternative to, or sometime substitute for, intercourse. If an individual or a couple can no longer enjoy intercourse as they once did because of either erectile problems, ejaculatory/orgasmic difficulties, or painful genital sensations, this does not mean it is no longer possible to feel close and give and receive pleasure.

For some people masturbation is an acceptable and satisfying alternative to intercourse. If a person is experiencing uncomfortable genital sensations or difficulty becoming sexually aroused, he or she may discover that sexual satisfaction is more easily and comfortably attained through self-stimulation than by trying to describe to a partner just what does or does not feel good. Masturbation can be a "successful," intimate, shared experience with a partner or a satisfying and relaxing experience when done alone.

Honest discussion of sexual feelings and activities is heartily encouraged. Some individuals find it difficult to talk about sexual topics, such as anatomy, variations of the sex act, or what feels good. Shared reading material can often be a very helpful introduction to frank discussion. Books or pamphlets can provide the vocabulary and visual images that many people may be too inhibited to use on their own.

SEXUAL DIFFICULTIES RELATING TO PHYSICAL CHANGES

Bodily changes that do not directly affect the sexual response can, however, interfere with a satisfactory sexual life. Fatigue may affect a person's level of sexual interest and make it difficult to initiate or carry on sexual activity. Individuals with MS frequently report that by evening, when the sexual partner is home and interested in having sex, they are just too tired to respond or enjoy it. It is helpful to remember that sexual activity is not a contest or an athletic marathon. It can continue to be a time of closeness, holding, sharing, and talking. If physical activity is possible and feels good, it is there to be enjoyed; otherwise partners can experiment with other ways of feeling pleasure and communicating loving feelings. The primary solution to the problem of fatigue is to conserve energy whenever possible. Use of a motorized wheelchair or cart (such as an Amigo or Portascoot) can relieve fatigue. Allowing for frequent rest periods during the course of the day is also beneficial. Making use of morning time for sexual activity, when most individuals with MS feel strongest, can maximize energy and interest levels. In addition, medication (such as Cylert, a central nervous system stimulant that is not an amphetamine and has few side effects) is sometimes helpful in the relief of lassitude and fatigue.

Weakness, pain, stiffness, spasticity, or contractures can make certain movements or positions difficult to achieve. At times it becomes impossible to find a comfortable position for satisfying sexual activities. Tremors or incoordination may make even the simplest or gentlest movements impossible or awkward. Medications and surgical procedures for these problems are discussed in Chapters 6 and 8.

In general, sexual interaction may be complicated by concerns about a variety of possible physical problems, including loss of bowel or bladder control, personal hygiene, pain, pressure sores, or urinary tract infections. Each partner may silently wonder to what extent the other harbors such concerns. The MS individual may feel fragile, uncertain, or even afraid of sexual contact. These feelings are easily transmitted to a partner who, in turn, holds back and feels anxious and inhibited. Here again, the ability to share these feelings with a partner leads to greater relaxation and intimacy. In fact, the intimacy and trust that is achieved through greater openness can replace some of what is lost in reduced sexual activity.

Couples frequently report that their sexual lives have become so encumbered that any chance at sexual spontaneity is lost. For a couple in which one partner is severely disabled, so much planning and arranging is required for sexual activity that it becomes difficult to feel relaxed, uninhibited, or spontaneous. Couples can learn to be creative in dealing with this particular kind of problem. First, to the extent that it is possible, nursing activities should be carried out by someone other than a family member so that the disabled partner can retain the role and feelings of being a partner rather than a patient. It is also important that a couple's bedroom not be turned into a sickroom. The reality in our culture is that illness and sexuality are not usually thought of together. It is easier to have sexual feelings when not surrounded by nursing equipment. Second, preparation for sexual activity can always be accompanied by intimate conversation, relaxing music, even a little wine if bladder control is not a problem. The preparation for sex becomes part of the sexual activity rather than a tiresome preamble. Third, it is extremely important for men and women with MS to continue to try to look and feel as attractive as they possibly can. The need for a catheter or a wheelchair should in no way lessen a person's need to be clean, stylish, and neat. A person who feels attractive will be more confident and more relaxed about sex and therefore more sexually attractive to his or her partner.

Loss of bladder or bowel control, or the use of a urinary catheter, can cause considerable inconvenience and anxiety to sexual partners. There is a two-step process involved in coping with this problem. First, it is necessary for people with MS to learn about bladder and bowel problems and their management. The medical and mechanical aspects of these symptoms are discussed fully in Chapter 11.

Bladder symptoms such as urgency and frequency of urination and incontinence are often relieved by some combination of the following: a modified fluid intake (especially during the few hours before going to bed), scheduling regular bowel movements, medication, and intermittent catheterization. Individuals must experiment, in collaboration with their doctor, until the most satisfactory solution is found. Although this process may take time and patience, successful bladder management is essential for good health and peace of mind, both of which are important ingredients in a satisfactory sex life. Urinary tract infections can result when the bladder is not properly managed. These infections are uncomfortable and require prompt medical attention, but they are *not* transmitted to a sexual partner.

Because of the degree of constipation experienced by most people with MS, bowel incontinence during sex is less likely to occur. In general, bowel incontinence is most effectively prevented with a carefully managed regimen of bowel evacuation several times weekly. The bowel management regimen can include modifications in diet, stool softeners, mild laxatives, suppositories, and, in the case of long-term intractable problems, enemas. The use of any of these measures should be reviewed with a physician.

The second step in bowel and bladder management is more difficult to achieve, for it involves ongoing openness and flexibility between sexual partners. Both partners need to be able to express their honest feelings about these problems. The feelings may include anxiety, anger, disgust, or inhibition of sexual arousal. Any and all of these emotional responses are normal, and couples need to be able to share them without feeling guilty. Being able to talk freely about these feelings will help to reduce their intensity. This will enable the partners to support each other more easily through any necessary changes or adjustments in their sex life.

PSYCHOLOGICAL CONFLICTS

Individuals coping with MS frequently experience marked changes in their feelings about themselves and their bodies. The disease, which can alter physical appearance and abilities, bodily functions, and activities of living, can also damage a person's self-image. These changes can easily affect one's sex life. The person who no longer sees him- or herself as healthy, active, or intact may have difficulty having sexual feelings or feeling sexually attractive. In our culture sex is closely associated with health and vigor. Sexual activities may at first seem incompatible with illness even if there is little disability.

Some individuals report that at times they feel remote from their own bodies, as though the disabled limbs could not possibly be part of them. In these instances the person's body image is not fully integrated with his or her physical state; the person may feel sexual or aroused but be unable to accept that disability and sex can go together.

Social changes that can occur with MS (such as unemployment, divorce, or increased dependence) may be reflected in a lowering of self-esteem, which in turn may contribute to sexual difficulties. Individuals, disabled or not, can experience sexual difficulties during periods when they do not feel good about themselves or their bodies. Self-esteem can also be affected by sexual performance; being able to perform satisfactorily in their sexual role plays an important part in determining how adult men and women feel about themselves. For many individuals, sexual gratification comes as much from "performing" well and pleasing a partner as it does from having an orgasm. People with MS and their partners frequently need to redefine what it means to "perform" well. Otherwise, they may become so worried about their ability to be adequate, attractive sexual partners that they shy away from intimate contact, convinced that they are no longer desirable.

In addition to changes in an individual's self-image and self-esteem, alterations frequently occur in interpersonal relationships. Three primary types of change are reported by families to cause a significant amount of stress: one is related to level of intimacy, another to gender roles, and the third to "caretaking" activities.

Couples who have been particularly close, functioning much like a team, frequently report that the MS acts like an intruder on their relationship. Confronted by something they are unable to share totally, each feels alienated and abandoned by the other. This inability to share may then intrude on their sexual intimacy as well.

For some families, traditional gender roles are highly valued and not easily changed. If the husband becomes unable to continue as breadwinner, or a wife cannot carry out her chosen activities inside and outside the home, these changes may be perceived as a loss of masculinity or femininity. The individuals may feel inadequate in their chosen roles, and this may carry over into their feelings about their sexual attractiveness. A spouse may also perceive the disabled partner as less masculine or feminine and therefore less attractive because of the alteration in roles.

The last type of role change involves the able-bodied spouse who becomes a nurse for the MS partner. It is very difficult for some individuals to respond sexually to a partner they have recently dressed, carried to the bathroom, catheterized, or cleaned.

Negative, angry feelings, a frequent accompaniment of the role changes described here, can also interfere with satisfying sexual activity. The able-bodied spouse may resent the changes brought about in the family by MS and be quite angry about the role changes forced on all of them. He or she may feel guilty about having these feelings toward the handicapped partner and be unable to express them. The MS partner can become very anxious and angry about his or her increased dependence and fearful of abandonment by the spouse on whom she has become dependent. Frequently individuals with MS report increasing resentment toward the spouse who nurses them, and they hesitate to express these feelings because of their fears of abandonment. These unspoken feelings in both partners can obviously impede the expression of positive loving feelings.

Couples who are experiencing sexual difficulties frequently report that they have also become less affectionate or demonstrative with each other. Most often, the satisfaction derived from close physical contact is lost because of anger or anxiety around sexual problems or other negative life changes brought about by MS. Resentment over changes in their sexual life and anxiety about the ability to perform or feel sexual can lead partners to pull away from one another. "If I can't have sex the way I used to, why bother?" is the kind of feeling that can develop. As a result, frustration over sexual problems is compounded by loneliness and a feeling of isolation.

Dealing with Psychological Factors

The psychological factors that interfere with sexual interest and performance (such as overwhelming depression or anger, reduced self-esteem, and anxiety about ability to perform) are relieved most effectively through psychotherapy. The therapy can occur on an individual basis or with couples or groups. The general applicability of psychotherapy for individuals with MS is reviewed in Chapter 13. Briefly, therapy helps persons with MS and their families acknowledge, mourn, and accept the losses imposed on their lives. In this ongoing process, depression, frustration, and anxiety are relieved, and the individuals learn how to cope more effectively, productively, and enjoyably with the everyday problems and unpredictability of MS.

Group therapy can be very helpful both for individuals who are part of a couple and those who are not. It offers the opportunity for peer support and the sharing of experiences and feelings. The most common themes around sexuality to emerge in groups include:

1. Can I still be sexually attractive to someone if I'm handicapped?
2. Is my sexuality determined by others' responses to me or by my feelings about myself? Does being handicapped make me less masculine or feminine?
3. Can I still be a satisfactory sex partner even if I can't perform as I used to or do not have the same level of sexual interest?
4. How will I deal with my sexual feelings if I do not have a sex partner?

Group members are usually quite relieved to discover that others share their problems and concerns. There is no one answer to any of these questions, and each individual develops his or her own answers within the supportive group setting.

In couples therapy pertaining to sexual problems, the partners are helped to talk more openly about their sexual interests and feelings (both loving and angry). The changes imposed by MS make it more important than usual for couples to be able to talk freely about what they want, what does or does not feel good, and what is sexually stimulating. Each partner needs to feel comfortable expressing these feelings and requests without fear of being criticized or abruptly rejected by the other. In the same way, each partner needs to feel free to say no—in a gentle and noncritical way—to requests or suggestions that are unappealing.

The emotional impact of MS may introduce worry, anxiety, or depression into daily living and into sexual interactions. These feelings can lead to temporary or long-term difficulties for any individual or couple. Communication between partners, which is more imperative in times of difficulty, often becomes impossible. Feelings of loss, anger, resentment, frustration, and uncertainty can burden both partners, rendering them unable or unwilling to be open about such problems.

It is important to emphasize that these feelings are common in even the most loving couples. The goal of couples' treatment is to bring the feelings out into the open, reassure the couple of the normality of these feelings, and help them to come to terms with the changes imposed on their relationship. If sexual intercourse ceases to be an option, this is a significant loss, which must be recognized and mourned. The couple who can share this loss openly will more likely continue sharing physical closeness and begin exploring and experimenting with alternative ways of expressing loving feelings and giving each other pleasure and comfort.

SOCIAL PRESSURE

The neurological, physical, and psychological problems that have been discussed here result from bodily changes or emotional reactions experienced by the person with MS. This section deals with the problems that result from the reactions and attitudes of others. Although these problems can affect anyone with MS, particular attention is paid to unmarried people who are not involved in a long-term relationship.

The current social attitudes toward health and sexuality may create special problems for the unmarried person with MS. Coping and communication may be particularly difficult; rather than having to learn how to work with one other person in coping with sexual problems, the single person may need to cope alone or with a series of people. A dating couple will probably not have the same commitment to each other or to the relationship as would a married couple. Although sexual problems can certainly cause significant stress or unhappiness for a married couple, there may be greater motivation to overcome or overlook them for the sake of preserving the family relationships. The unmarried individual, on the other hand, may fear that a successful, intimate relationship can never begin or continue.

Three questions are commonly asked by single men and women with MS:

1. "How do I meet people if I can't participate in many of the social activities that other singles enjoy?"
2. "Who will want to get involved in a long-term relationship with me and this disease?"
3. "When should I tell the other person about my MS?"

The major significance of these questions is that they are asked at one time or another by almost all MS patients. The answers to these questions vary tremendously from one individual to another.

Physical disability may indeed interfere with a person's chances of making social contacts at a singles' bar or sports event. People whose choice of recreation primarily involves sports or other strenuous physical activity are not as likely to be attracted to someone who cannot participate in these activities as are people whose interests are less physical. There are, however, other ways of meeting people. Taking classes, joining clubs or religious organizations, pursuing one's career, or doing volunteer work are all ways in which many people with MS have found satisfying relationships. The important thing seems to be to participate in group activities that are not physically taxing and in which it is possible to become an active, contributing member. This gives others the opportunity to get acquainted and comfortable with a person apart from his or her disability. Discussion and support groups for the handicapped, such as those sponsored by many MS Society chapters, not only provide an opportunity for meeting people but also enable men and women to share ideas on how to meet others.

There is no doubt that the problems and uncertainties of MS will cause some potential partners to shy away from a long-term relationship. This will not be true of everyone, however. The disabled person too often falls into the trap of saying, "Why should I try to meet anyone—who would want me anyway?" In other words, the person anticipates a negative response from others rather than taking a chance and waiting to see what happens. He or she withdraws from people and activities in order to avoid disappointment. A certain amount of unhappiness and rejection is unavoidable—as is true for anyone—so the best course may be for the handicapped individual to let others get to know and like him/her and then make their own decision. This will occur most successfully in those kinds of group activities in which MS interferes least.

How and when to tell others about the MS seems to be a difficult issue for many people. On the one hand, MS plays a significant role in one's life and emotions. It is difficult to lay the groundwork for a satisfying, meaningful relationship while hiding such an important aspect of one's life. On the other hand, many people fear that talking about MS will cause the other person to run away before the relationship can even begin. There is no one correct solution to this dilemma, and each person must eventually sort it out for him- or herself. Sharing one's feelings about this issue with others who are handicapped can be reassuring; it helps the person to feel less alone with the problem and provides a chance to learn from others' experiences. The most important rule of thumb is that no two people respond to another's disability in exactly the same way. One or two rejections do not mean that another will necessarily follow.

For the severely disabled person, finding sexual partners can indeed be a significant problem. The person may be sexually interested but feel unattractive to potential partners. The feeling that one is unattractive, although often unwarranted and unrealistic, may nevertheless be strong. A disabled person who is unsuccessful with one sexual partner may become convinced that no one will ever again find him/her attractive. The unfortunate reality is that our culture places great value on youth and health in relation to sexuality. Given that this is so, the very disabled individual may indeed not be as sexually attractive to others as a nondisabled person might be. He or she may then need to deal with this loss and find alternatives, either in the form of increased individual sexual activities such as masturbation or other interesting and satisfying nonsexual activities. Companionship and the sharing of common interests need not be lost simply because one is not involved in a sexual relationship. People who have a variety of interests and enjoy sharing them will always be valued by others. The challenge lies in finding practical and enjoyable ways of pursuing these activities, hobbies, or talents.

An additional word should be said about the possible problems confronted by gay men and women who have MS. They have great difficulty in finding help with sexual questions, either in the literature on disability, which tends to ignore the problems and needs of gay people, or from health professionals who may shy away from any issues related to homosexuality. Being a "minority within a minority" can make it doubly difficult to find the help and support one needs in dealing with sexual or any other kinds of problems. Gay men and women will need to confront these difficulties head on if they are to find the support they need. Therapists, sex counselors, and health professionals who are comfortable with, and knowledgeable about, sexual difficulties, disability, and homosexuality can be found. Again, finding one unhelpful or rejecting professional does not mean that all will be that way.

CHILDBEARING AND BIRTH CONTROL

Fertility remains for the most part unimpaired in individuals with MS. Couples engaging in intercourse must make the same decisions about birth control as do individuals without neurological impairment. Any form of birth control that is effective and manageable is permitted with MS. Some women with weakness or tremor in the hands find the diaphragm to be cumbersome. Similarly, men with dexterity problems find it difficult to put on a condom. Such problems can be solved by having the partner insert the diaphragm or put on the condom as part of the sexual foreplay. Where such a solution is not practical or desirable, birth control pills are usually an acceptable means of birth control.

The decision of whether to have children is a very personal one. There is no medical reason why an adult with MS should not become a parent. Multiple sclerosis has not been shown to cause miscarriages, birth defects, or impaired fertility. An otherwise healthy young woman with MS should not have trouble conceiving and delivering a normal infant.

The effects of pregnancy on MS are variable. Most of the scientific studies that have been done in this area support the conclusion that pregnancy has no deleterious effect on long-term disability in women with MS. Patients who become pregnant have been shown to have a lower risk of exacerbations during pregnancy and a slightly higher risk of exacerbations in the 3 to 6 months after the baby is born.

Multiple sclerosis patients may find that some preexisting symptoms may become worse temporarily during pregnancy. These include fatigue, urinary frequency, or constipation. As the uterus enlarges, and the patient's center of gravity shifts, ambulation may be impeded, and patients may have to use aids such as canes, walkers, or wheelchair during pregnancy to help them ambulate and avoid the danger of falling. Bowel and bladder hygiene may be adjusted to accommodate the problems posed by an enlarged uterus pressing on the bladder.

The decision of whether or not an MS patient should have children should take into consideration emotional, financial, and family support considerations as well as medical questions. Many MS patients say that having children has enriched their lives and outweighs any disadvantages.

SUMMARY

It is clear that sexual problems related to MS can take many forms and affect many areas of the sexual relationship. These problems are compounded by the difficulties individuals and couples have in discussing their concerns with each other and their doctors. We hope that this chapter will serve to reassure a person with MS that he or she is not alone with these problems. The knowledgeable health care professional or family or sex therapist is available to provide help and support with this adjustment. Likewise, spouse, lover, or friends may be crucial. Sexual feelings and their enjoyment can continue to be an important part of living and relating even if the mode of sexual expression requires some adjustment.

13

Psychological Issues

Nicholas G. LaRocca, Rosalind C. Kalb, and Seymour R. Kaplan

Compared to diseases that were well known in antiquity, MS is relatively new. Writings of the period indicate that Saint Lidwina of Schiedam (1380–1433) suffered from MS. Augustus D'Este (1794–1848), grandson of George III of England, recorded his MS symptoms in a richly detailed diary. The earliest scientific descriptions of the disease appeared in 1835. In 1868, the French neuropsychiatrist Jean Charcot, a teacher of Freud, described the relationship between MS and scarred lesions distributed throughout the white matter of the central nervous system. Charcot's name for the disease, *sclerose en plaques* or sclerosis in plaques, survives in English as "multiple sclerosis," meaning many scars.

Multiple sclerosis has long been the subject of psychological research and conjecture. In his diary, Augustus D'Este described the onset of symptoms shortly after the death of a beloved father figure. Charcot also observed that grief or anger might precipitate the disease. During the late 19th century hysteria was a subject of intense study in Europe by Charcot, Freud, Breuer, and others. Partly because of the close resemblance of many of their symptoms (e.g., paresthesias, visual loss, difficulty walking), hysteria and MS were thought to be related. In addition, the frequent appearance of euphoria, depression, emotional lability, and intellectual decline in people with MS further stimulated interest in the psychological aspects of this disease.

In those early years scientific interest in MS was most pronounced in North America and Europe. Two schools of thought arose concerning the psychological aspects of MS. In the English-speaking world it was widely believed that certain personality types were MS-prone, especially in the face of emotional distress. The contrasting school of thought, most prominent in France and Germany, held that the psychological phenomena seen in MS (e.g., euphoria, depression, intellectual change) were either direct results of the disease or were reactions to the real-life effects of the illness. We can call these two schools of thought the stress–illness model (emotional stress leads to illness) and the illness–stress model (the illness leads to emotional stress).

STRESS–ILLNESS

Many of the early studies of psychological aspects of MS were psychoanalytically oriented. They found a high degree of psychiatric disorder among MS patients, especially hysterical personality patterns. These findings crystallized into the concept of the MS-prone personality, allegedly an immature, dependent, and hysterical pattern. This concept reached its fullest development in the United States, where prevailing psychosomatic theory held that specific personality patterns caused specific illnesses. Disease was the combined result of specific organ vulnerability, a predisposing personality pattern, and an emotional precipitant. The precipitating event (e.g., death of a loved one) mobilized a central conflict specific to the vulnerable organ while stripping away the primary defenses against the conflict.

In MS, it was thought that emotional conflict arising from oedipal fixations led to vascular changes in the brain. These vascular changes were thought to cause the demyelination that in turn led to MS symptoms. Psychotherapy was actually recommended at one time as a preventive measure for susceptible personalities. Researchers sought in vain for some specific personality pattern that preceded the onset of MS. However, evidence to date suggests that all types of personalities get MS and that there is no MS-prone personality.

As the notion of the MS-prone personality has faded, increasing attention has been paid to the other part of the equation, the emotional precipitant. Current thinking has thus turned from the search for a specific personality pattern causing MS to the identification of nonspecific psychological factors that might contribute to the development of illness. Emotional stress is the factor that has received the most attention.

Returning to Augustus D'Este and Charcot, we find that stress has long been regarded as a precipitant of both the onset of MS and subsequent attacks. This idea received international attention in 1979 when Richard Queen, a U.S. State Department employee, developed MS symptoms during his protracted captivity by Iranians at the American Embassy in Teheran.

Since 1950, 11 published studies have addressed the role of stress in MS disease activity. Of these, seven used the case-study method, examining a sample of MS patients with no control group. Four used the case-control method, comparing a sample of MS patients with a control group consisting either of patients with other medical conditions or persons with no medical problems. Although the results of the case studies tended to favor a stress–MS link, the case-control studies have been evenly divided. Thus, considering the existing research as a whole, results have been inconclusive, and the role of stress as a precipitant of disease activity in MS remains unclear.

If stress does play a role in MS, it is probably a minor role, operating in conjunction with biological factors such as a slow virus and/or an autoimmune response (Chapter 3). In other words, when the physical conditions for the development of the disease already exist, stress may increase the likelihood that the individual will develop the disease. In people who already have MS, stress may slightly increase the frequency and severity of exacerbations (flare-ups of the disease). Scientific evidence for such effects is very sketchy at present. More research is needed to determine if stress plays a role in MS. In the meantime, stress should be regarded as a normal feature of living. Many useful strategies exist for coping with stress (such as hypnosis, relaxation, meditation, and biofeedback). Although there is no proof that stress management techniques have any effect on MS, they do contribute to a sense of well-being and are generally harmless. Certainly no one with MS should attempt to manage stress by avoiding stressful situations altogether—that could mean renouncing life almost completely.

ILLNESS–STRESS

As we have seen, evidence concerning the possible psychological precipitants of MS is inconclusive. The contrasting point of view, that MS leads to a number of psychological consequences, will now be examined. This school of thought, at one time more prominent in Europe, looked on intellectual change, euphoria, emotional lability, depression, etc. as possible manifestations of damage to the central nervous system.

Intellectual Changes

Although American authorities in the early 20th century tended to deemphasize its importance, intellectual change was early recognized as a possible result of MS. Controversy has long surrounded this issue. Even today it is difficult to state with any certainty the frequency, nature, and severity of intellectual changes in MS. Modern estimates of the frequency of such changes range from 25 to 65% of all MS patients. Given current evidence, it is quite likely that approximately 45 to 55% of people with MS have some intellectual deficits that can be measured using specialized psychological tests.

The prevailing view is that most such changes are subtle. A small number, perhaps only 5 to 10% of all patients, have changes severe enough to limit their everyday functioning. Compared to weakness, incoordination, fatigue, and visual problems, intellectual change is an infrequent cause of limitation in the life of the person with MS.

Since demyelination can occur in any of the brain's many areas of white matter, a variety of functions may be affected. Although there is incomplete agreement concerning the specific abilities affected, the ones most frequently cited are memory for recent events, abstract reasoning, verbal fluency ("it's on the tip of my tongue" phenomenon), judgment, and most spatial and motor abilities.

These problems are generally thought to be more likely to appear as the disease progresses and to worsen slowly over time. Evidence for this is tentative at best, and there certainly exist large numbers of MS patients with very advanced disease and perfectly intact intellectual functioning.

Euphoria

Even before the turn of the century, euphoria had been described in MS. Later, this exaggerated or inappropriate sense of well-being came to be regarded as characteristic of the disease and generally accompanied by intellectual deterioration. For this reason it was believed to be a direct result of demyelination. Today euphoria seems to be less frequently observed than in Charcot's time. Clinicians still believe that euphoria is associated with advanced disease and intellectual decline, though there has been almost no research to confirm this.

Emotional Lability

Along with euphoria, emotional lability was one of the first psychological changes to be described in MS. In its more severe manifestations, lability consists of uncontrollable fits of laughing and crying that have little or nothing to do with how a person is actually feeling. This change is thought to be caused by demyelination in fibers running between the brainstem, located at the base of the skull, and the higher structures of the brain. Although generally regarded as uncommon, lability has generated increased interest of late as a result of the report of successful treatment with antidepressant medication.

The MS Personality

Around the same time that some researchers were searching for the specific personality pattern that caused MS, others were looking for the personality produced by the disease. The presence of euphoria and lability, along with the confusion between hysteria and MS, encouraged such research. It was thought that MS produced a characteristic psychiatric disorder. This belief reflected the prevailing view that adjustment to chronic illness generally took the form of psychopathology and could be understood by using the same methods employed in assessing psychiatric illness. Not surprisingly, the results of such studies were inconsistent, since adjustment to chronic illness is a process of growth and change, to which each individual brings his or her own emotional strengths and weaknesses.

Adjustment as a Model

In recent years, the assumption that the stress of MS produced an MS personality or some form of mental illness has been replaced by a new set of assumptions concerning how people adjust to a pervasive and long-standing stressor. First, adjustment to MS, with all its emotional upheaval, is seen as a normal human response to a catastrophic stress, which in very few cases results in psychiatric illness. Second, adjustment is the result of a host of factors including characteristics of the disease, the individual, and the cultural and social context. How well a person adjusts is thus determined by the interplay of many forces. Third, adjustment is not a single event but a life-long process that is in a constant state of flux.

What We Know

Having traced the evolution of the illness–stress model to the present, we find that MS may be regarded as a major and generally permanent life stressor, adjustment to which emerges as the major psychological issue of interest. What do we know to date concerning how people adjust to this stressor?

1. There is no "MS personality." People with MS do have many experiences in common as a result of the illness but do not share any particular personality pattern.

2. Although periodic psychological distress is very much a part of MS, it generally does not take the form of psychiatric illness.

3. Depression and/or grief is a frequent experience of people with MS. Grief seems to be especially significant, as people with MS go through a process of mourning for losses brought on by the illness. There are probably many different psychological states in MS, all currently referred to as depression. Some of these may be grief, some may represent personality changes directly caused by brain lesions, and others may be depressive disorders predating the MS. Further research is needed if we are fully to understand the wide array of MS experiences that at present all go by the catch-all of depression.

4. Psychotherapeutic interventions can alleviate depression in some individuals with MS.

5. Psychological distress frequently increases when exacerbations occur and may abate with time or when there is a remission. In contrast, such distress may bear little or no relationship to the severity of the disability.

6. Although self-esteem may be seriously challenged by MS-related life changes, it seems to be very resilient. People with MS generally have levels of self-esteem that do not differ greatly from those of the general population.

7. Knowing more about the illness seems to help many individuals in the adjustment process.

With the illness–stress model in mind, let us examine in greater detail the psychological issues confronted by the person diagnosed with MS. For the purpose of clarity and simplicity, the person with MS will be referred to as "she" simply because the ratio of female to male patients is approximately 1.7 : 1.

THE EMOTIONAL CHALLENGES OF MS

Dealing with the Diagnosis: An Adjustment Process

The psychological stress of MS begins even before the diagnosis is made. The person may experience puzzling and distressing symptoms for months—or even years—before they are correctly identified. One study found that an average of 3 years passed between the onset of symptoms and the communication of the diagnosis to the patient. Friends, relatives, and doctors may even suggest that the symptoms are imaginary, leaving the person to cope alone with physical discomfort and emotional distress. A great deal of time and money may be expended in the effort to find a name for the symptoms.

Once the physician has used the appropriate tests to determine the diagnosis (see Chapter 4), the person should be given this information. Some health care professionals withhold the diagnosis or give some euphemistic label (e.g., "demylinating disease" or "virus of the nervous system") in order to spare themselves or their patients the stress of dealing with multiple sclerosis. Until the patient has a name for the problem, however, she cannot even begin the long adjustment process.

Individuals react in very different ways to hearing the diagnosis. "I've never heard of MS"; "Thank God it's not cancer"; "I knew I wasn't crazy"; "Why me?" are some of the more common responses, indicating a mixture of acute distress and bittersweet relief. Whatever the person's initial response, however, she must begin to grieve. Grief seems to be the necessary initial step in the adjustment process. Even if the person is not disabled, she has been told that there is something wrong and must begin to see herself differently. This means the loss of her old self-image and the development of a somewhat altered one. Any loss of this type requires grieving.

It is important for health care professionals and family members to help the newly diagnosed person acknowledge and experience these feelings of grief. She may not even recognize this as the source of the painful feelings. The normal, expectable grief reaction to the diagnosis may include crying, reminiscing about a less painful past, expressing strong feelings of rage, resentment, and fear, or even massive denial that there is any problem at all.

Normal grieving may continue for several months, and it will recur intermittently as the person experiences changes in her condition or increased disability. If, however, the person's grief reaction continues unabated for more than a year, the reaction may be more problematic. In a "pathological grief reaction," the person may become totally hopeless about the future, unable to enjoy any aspect of her life, or emotionally rigid to the point of being unable to make even minor life adjustments. Additional signs include sleeplessness and loss of appetite over a prolonged period and the inability to participate productively or enjoyably in work or leisure activities. As will be discussed in greater detail, this type of grief reaction requires professional intervention and usually responds well to group and individual counseling.

Family Upheaval

If and when the person with MS experiences greater disability and reduced mobility, she may begin to discover that she can no longer meet some of her own expectations or the expectations of others. At this time troublesome patterns can begin to emerge within the family.

Overinvolvement in Disability

It may, for example, be difficult for family members to accommodate to the fact that only one of them is disabled. Activities that were once enjoyed by the family as a whole are given up by all. Thus, for example, a family used to taking family ski trips may give up skiing altogether, often resulting in unspoken feelings of sadness, guilt, and resentment. Or a husband may continue to play in weekly bowling tournaments even though his wife can no longer participate. Although this is often a very healthy and necessary course to follow, many painful feelings can emerge. The wife may feel jealous and resentful while the husband feels guilty over his need to retain a "normal" life-style. Family members need to talk openly about these feelings so that everyone's emotional needs can be met. This kind of honest sharing begins the creative problem-solving process needed to find satisfying alternatives. These satisfying alternatives will enable families to remain intact through the stresses imposed by the disease.

Loss of Partnership

If the person with MS becomes severely disabled, she and her spouse may begin to experience a painful shift in their personal relationship. She may resent being made to feel more and more like a child while her husband has to assume the nursing role. He grieves over the loss of a "partner" and resents the burdens of caretaking. In this kind of situation, the partner with MS is afraid to express her resentment for fear of being abandoned, while the spouse feels too guilty to complain. Again, it is only through the open sharing of these feelings that partners can minimize the upheaval in their personal relationship.

The Able-Bodied as an Extension of the Disabled

At times the severely disabled partner may become quite bossy in her requests for help—"Bring me that book," or "Pick up that paper." These requests are not meant to be imperious but are simply delivered as if she were telling her own arms and legs what to do. Unfortunately, the able-bodied spouse at the receiving end of these commands may begin to feel more like an appendage of his wife than a separate person. To protect his personal space and identity, he refuses, and a pattern of frustration and resentment is established for them both. When couples begin to recognize the feelings of frustration and impotence that lead to these commands, this pattern can be halted. The disabled partner can recognize her spouse's need for some uninterrupted time and space, and the spouse can more easily comprehend the urgency behind her request.

Role Confusion

The children of a disabled parent may become very anxious when caretaking roles become altered or reversed. Expecting mother to take care of them, they suddenly find themselves having to take care of her. They may feel the need to test the limits within the family structure in order to determine who is really in charge. This kind of misbehaving can be frightening to everyone including themselves. A disabled parent often needs help in developing new and different parenting skills so that she can convey to her children a continuing sense of security and safety.

These are some of the problematic patterns that sometimes develop within the family. Being aware of potential problems can make it easier to recognize and discuss them openly with all family members. When and if communication becomes too difficult, a family therapist can provide support while helping each family member to understand the others' needs.

Although the changes imposed by MS can precipitate the kinds of problems described here, it is helpful to remember that they also provide the opportunity for satisfying growth. On their own, or with the help of a therapist, family members can achieve greater understanding and sensitivity, develop new interests, and share a satisfying sense of unity as they deal with the challenges of MS.

Anxiety: The Result of Feeling Out of Control

The cause, course, and outcome of multiple sclerosis are all uncertain, with the result that the person never knows what tomorrow will bring.

Daily confrontations with the unknown frequently result in anxiety. This kind of "anticipatory anxiety" is a common reaction to the unpredictability of MS.

Occasional loss of bladder or bowel control is one of the clearest precipitants of this type of anxiety. The person with bladder or bowel problems anxiously awaits some catastrophe to occur, whether it be during a business meeting, social event, or sexual activity. Such a prospect threatens her feelings of control, of independence, and of being an adult. At times, the anxiety becomes more disabling than the disease, and the person refuses to leave home.

Help for this type of anxiety comes from two primary sources. First, the person can discuss bladder/bowel problems openly with her physician and learn effective self-management techniques (see Chapter 11). In this way she regains a sense of control over her own body and revives her feelings of independence and maturity. The second important source of support comes from other people with MS. Participation in group counseling is particularly helpful because it enables the person to share her feelings with other men and women who are coping with similar experiences. As a result she no longer feels so different or alone.

Support for efforts to cope with the more general unpredictability of the disease is also found in the group setting. Group members can help each other to recognize options and live life fully while at the same time preparing for possible problems and changes. This kind of shared coping and planning does much to heighten feelings of control and reduce anxiety.

Loss of Self-Esteem

If the person's MS continues to progress, her ability to carry out valued roles may be impaired. She may be unable to function in her chosen career or carry out her domestic responsibilities. When a person can no longer perform at a level that meets her own standards and expectations, she experiences a loss of self-esteem. This loss results from the feeling that she is no longer the person she thought she was or thinks she ought to be.

Faced with the necessity of redefining or reorganizing her major life roles, the person needs support in her efforts to find meaningful and creative alternatives. The support can come from family and friends, health care professionals, or others with MS. With this support she will be able to make the changes and adjustments that are required of her while continuing to feel good about herself. Thus, for example, a woman who has valued her ability to cook elaborate meals for family and guests may need to discover alternative ways of expressing this creative nurturance. A man who has used sports activities as a way of interacting with his children may need to experiment with other forms of play and communication. Similarly, a person whose career choice has involved a great deal of physical activity may need to discover and cultivate other talents and interests. The need to alter one's goals or one's life-style can involve both painful loss and exciting challenge. A person faced with the necessity of abandoning a career or altering any other major life role is forced to look within herself for satisfying alternatives. People often report that the misfortune of MS has forced them to become acquainted with strengths, talents, and interests they never knew they had.

INTERVENTION

The Value of Intermittent Psychological Support

It is clear that the emotional challenge of MS is great. At the present time, there is neither a cure for MS nor a totally satisfactory treatment. What is available, however, is a variety of tools and strategies that can be used to cope with the demands of the disease. As described in this book these tools include mechanical support devices, drugs for symptomatic relief, techniques for bladder/bowel control, and strategies for conservation of time and energy. Psychological counseling by a mental health professional is another valuable tool.

For many, "counseling" is still perceived as an activity for the unstable or the emotionally weak. It is considered a "cop out" or an invasion of privacy. Some people with MS interpret the wish or need for counseling as a sign that they are disabled emotionally as well as physically. To counter these misconceptions, we propose an alternative view of counseling.

The physical and emotional demands of MS are ongoing. From the onset of the initial symptoms, the person with MS experiences some degree of uncertainty, anxiety, change, and loss. These feelings wax and wane, but they are always superimposed on the normal, everyday stresses and strains of living. Life is complex and problematic to us all, so it seems reasonable to expect that a person who must also deal with MS might at times feel frightened, bewildered, and alone. It is useful then to provide the person who has MS with the tools necessary for coping with these periods of extra stress and turmoil. These tools can be conceptualized as "intermittent psychological support."

In order to understand how the person with MS might benefit from this support, it is necessary to describe its various forms, such as orientation/information groups and individual, group, and family counseling. Although descriptions of these different forms of psychological support can overlap, there are specific uses for each of them.

Orientation/Information Groups

By the time MS is diagnosed, an individual may have had puzzling and uncomfortable symptoms for quite some time. Some people delay consulting a physician for fear of what they will hear, whereas others encounter physicians who are reluctant to communicate the diagnosis. In either case, the MS person is already experiencing significant stress and anxiety by the time the diagnosis is made. Under these circumstances, it may be very difficult to comprehend what the diagnosing physician is saying and even more difficult to think of important questions to ask.

Short-term orientation groups (8–10 sessions) conducted by health care professionals can provide people who have just received a diagnosis of MS with a relaxed setting in which to obtain information, ask questions, and feel less alone. People can obtain reading materials and information on available resources. They meet others who are newly diagnosed without having to encounter people who are more severely disabled. Most importantly, the orientation group can help people feel that it is acceptable to talk about the illness, even if they are not ready to do so right away. This lays the groundwork for future communication and support. Then, should the need arise at some future time, the person will find it easier to ask for help.

Individual Counseling

The process of "adjusting" to multiple sclerosis is not a simple, one-time event. For each individual, adjustment gradually evolves during the course of the disease. At various points along the way, an individual might experience enough stress to feel the need for additional emotional support. There are three situations in which individual counseling with a mental health professional can be particularly helpful.

Individual counseling is recommended for the individual whose normal and necessary grief reaction to the diagnosis develops into depression. When the person with MS becomes depressed, he or she may experience the loss of control over certain aspects of daily living as a total loss of control. Life may then feel hopelessly frightening and empty. Under these circumstances, counseling facilitates healthy grieving, provides comfort and support, and helps the individual regain a sense of control through a recognition of available options.

A second situation in which individual counseling may be appropriate is when the emotional stress of MS accentuates preexisting problems to the extent that they no longer appear manageable. People usually find that in addition to the problems created by disability, the stress of adjustment also heightens conflicts that were already present in the individual or in the family. For example, a man who has always experienced a lack of self-confidence and a fear of failure might find the onset of physical disability both terrifying and guilt provoking. A woman with low self-esteem who has always relied on her physical appearance for her sense of worth may be particularly devastated by the diagnosis of a chronic disease. Individual counseling can help people identify the relationship between the MS and earlier fears and conflicts and perhaps resolve them.

Individual counseling can also be a helpful and necessary introduction to group counseling. Many who would benefit immensely from supportive contact with others with MS are initially reluctant to join a group. They fear people who are more disabled than they are and resent those who are less disabled. They feel frightened and alone and are reluctant to listen to other people's problems and fears when their own loom so large. Short-term individual counseling can reduce the individual's natural fear of others and help the MS person feel less desperate. He or she is then able to benefit from sharing the experience of a group.

Group Counseling

It is through the company of their peers that people most often find the help and support they need. Sharing experiences with others who understand or who have "been there" is a valuable way of finding answers and coming to terms with painful feelings. The benefits of group counseling under professional leadership are numerous, but among the most important are the following:

1. People can help one another identify career options, explore solutions to everyday problems, and recognize self-defeating attitudes or behaviors.
2. Group members can help each other recognize when and if they are "using" their disability to avoid responsibilities.
3. Group counseling also provides a setting in which adults can share their common anxieties about disability, loss of bowel or bladder control, and impotence without having to feel like children. People find that they are able to laugh about problems they thought they would never even be able to mention out loud.
4. Within the group, individuals can express feelings of anger, resentment, jealousy, or fear that might alienate or frighten family members or friends.
5. The group setting can provide a weekly respite from the strenuous daily efforts of coping in the able-bodied world.
6. Relationships formed in the group often continue long after group participation is over, providing a valuable social support network.

Group counseling can be beneficial to people who share common feelings or concerns. In addition to MS groups, there are groups for those whose spouses have been diagnosed as having MS, for children with a disabled parent, or for couples where one partner is disabled.

Family Counseling

While MS changes the life of the person who has the disease, it also affects the lives of family members. The stress of MS creates new problems in the family network and also heightens existing conflicts and problems. A family may find that it needs help in resolving problems that had seemed relatively manageable before the onset of the disease. In addition, the family may begin to experience the painful feelings and conflicts described earlier. Family counseling sessions can identify such situations before they reach the crisis point. The sessions provide a setting in which family members can learn to understand and accommodate each other's feelings and needs.

All of these forms of counseling can be incorporated into the concept of "intermittent psychological support." During any period of major change or stress, one or more forms of counseling may be utilized to provide information, support, and insight into feelings or problems. Different individuals make use of counseling in different ways, whether for a few months following the diagnosis or on a more long-term basis. Occasional sessions of individual or family counseling during periods of crisis are also valuable. In any of these situations, the goal is not to "find a cure" but to regain a sense of control over one's life. When a person feels overwhelmed by loss, anxiety, or change, it is difficult to recognize available options and make satisfying choices. Counseling is a tool that can help make this possible in a number of ways over the course of the disease.

CONCLUSION

Adjusting to MS means adjusting to an illness with many faces. Some of these faces are easier to deal with than others. Adjustment begins with the need to resolve the uncertainty produced by the first appearance of symptoms. Once a diagnosis is made, acceptance of the reality of having MS and all it implies can take place. Adaptation follows as the person with MS grieves for what has been lost and builds a new and different way of life. Once adaptation has occurred, MS may fade into the background a bit as the person with MS carries on the business of living.

The process of adjustment is affected by an individual's own coping ability, by aspects of the environment, and by characteristics of the disease. No two people adjust in the same way or at the same pace. Nevertheless, adjustment can be very successful, and the quality of life can remain quite good in spite of the tremendous challenges presented by MS.

14

Social Adaptations

Nancy J. Holland and Seymour R. Kaplan

The diagnosis of a chronic disease necessitates varying degrees of adaptive changes in all areas of living. Social adaptation to MS involves the assessment and possible readjustment of life-style, role expectations, and goals. This process can be difficult and confusing as the uncertainty of MS creates potential obstacles to every decision. Despite these difficulties, people living with MS need to examine important relationships, explore their options, and identify those situations where personal control can be exerted. The intent of this chapter is to increase awareness of areas to be explored and to encourage constructive planning.

A few points should be noted before proceeding. Psychological factors and responses (such as depression) overlap in many ways with social or relationship issues. These are discussed in Chapter 13. Likewise, sexuality is an important component of intimate relationships, and discussion of this area is concentrated in Chapter 12. Finally, many broad guidelines are stated here. It is well to remember that they are generalizations and so are not "right" for everyone. Thus, they are best approached as ideas for consideration, not as directives. The individual with MS, or a family member, must be the ultimate determinant of his or her attitudes and actions.

INTERPERSONAL RELATIONSHIPS

Individuals with MS generally experience anxiety about interpersonal relationships at some point following diagnosis. To tell or not to tell, how and when to tell, what information to communicate—these questions pertain not only to the newly diagnosed but to the majority of people with MS who have minimal visible dysfunction. Family members have similar concerns but may have emotional responses that are different from those of the person with MS such as guilt about good health or anger at life changes imposed by the chronic disease. These and other commonly encountered interpersonal difficulties are addressed in this section.

THE NEWLY DIAGNOSED PATIENT

Following diagnosis, much psychic energy is concentrated on integrating this new and frightening entity into one's concept of self. The impulse may be to inform everyone—an attempt to control reality by controlling the information communicated. Conversely, some people try to make MS "go away" by not discussing it with anyone. Neither extreme is helpful, and middle-ground responses can be achieved. In addition, both the MS individual and family feel frightened, sad, angry, or optimistic, but not necessarily in concert with each other. Dealing with this range of emotions while continuing with normal activities of daily living can only be described as very difficult and stressful. Although each situation is different and must be evaluated independently, some guidelines formulated from ongoing counseling with MS clients may be useful.

1. *Sharing information and feelings about a new MS diagnosis with "significant others"* (spouse, parents, roommate) generally releases pent-up emotions, relieves some feelings of aloneness, and allows those closest to be involved. Strong feelings are rarely effectively concealed, and the attempt to do so may alienate those with whom a loving and trusting relationship already exists.

2. *General disclosure to peripheral people* tends to increase anxiety at this point because repeated explanations are needed, and the fear of rejection usually accompanies each announcement. Also, the response of casual acquaintances may be more curiosity than concern. The emotional turbulence present following diagnosis makes such indiscriminate disclosure especially problematic.

3. *Grieving* is expected following diagnosis of a chronic illness such as MS. Spouses or others with a close emotional relationship may undergo a similar response. Communication during this time helps both parties and can actually strengthen the relationship.

4. *For those involved in dating situations,* disclosure of MS best occurs after a comfortable rapport has been established. This may be the first meeting or the tenth—whenever the relationship progresses toward emotional intimacy. Fear of the partner's response does not disappear or even diminish with time, as potential rejection is painful under any circumstances. Therefore, waiting for a totally comfortable moment will undoubtedly prolong anxiety within the relationship.

5. *Plans for the future* can be made optimistically, as most people with MS do not become severely disabled. However, "plan for the worst—hope for the best" is a good maxim to follow. For example, consider potential disability when a move to a new home is being planned. The need for structural accessibility may never materialize; but should disability occur, environmental barriers in the home will be one less problem with which to contend.

6. *Pregnancy* is not believed to affect the course of MS, and MS is not hereditary. Family planning can be guided by preexisting criteria, with some attention to the possible future disability of the MS parent.

7. *Gaining greater understanding of MS* by reading relevant material and questioning experienced health professionals usually increases the sense of control over the disease. Reducing the unknown to a known entity usually reduces the fear.

8. *When one becomes aware of the MS, most individuals and families experience varied and intense emotional responses.* They may perceive some of these feelings as being "bad" or "negative," depending on their upbringing and value systems. It is important for all concerned to understand that feelings themselves are neither good nor bad in the moral sense, although some are undeniably pleasant, whereas others are extremely painful. Moral judgment implies choice, whereas feelings simply emerge unsolicited by the individual. If feelings could be chosen, it is likely that joy and contentment would be prime selections. This concept is crucial when dealing with the emotional upheaval following an MS diagnosis, as feelings such as anger and depression are normal,

appropriate, and understandable. Difficulties arise when feelings such as these are denied or misdirected, particularly because the obvious target is loved ones. Try to talk openly with someone close about the feelings as they occur and why you may be experiencing them. This not only creates some control over the feelings through understanding, but such sharing with a loved one can lead to deepening of trust and affection between partners. It is important for the MS person/family to realize the influence they have over their relationships with others. People respond to unspoken cues—are you uncomfortable, self-conscious, defensive? An attitude that conveys that MS is an unpleasant fact of life but not consuming or unmentionable will help others relate in a natural and helpful way. How friends, coworkers and relatives respond to MS can be very much influenced by the messages the MS person and family communicate to other people.

9. *A comfortable, trusting relationship with a physician knowledgeable about MS* who is willing to deal with the varied and long-term manifestations of this chronic disease is invaluable. Many questions will arise requiring professional response. Complications can be anticipated and reduced or prevented by an alert and concerned physician. It is preferable to be involved with a doctor who works within an interdisciplinary or team setting, as various health professionals may be needed at different times. Communication between these professionals enhances and reinforces individualized care. This type of center is not available to most people, and so an appropriate "solo" practitioner is selected. This may be the family doctor, internist, or neurologist. Be sure that questions are answered satisfactorily and that follow-up appointments are scheduled. "Come back when you have a problem" often results in the recognition of problems after they have progressed needlessly.

10. *Counseling can be extremely helpful* during the period following establishment of the MS diagnosis. Although some people associate counseling or psychotherapy with mental illness or character weakness, anyone undergoing an unusual emotional stress, such as that imposed by MS, may benefit from psychological services. An objective, concerned mental health professional can help clarify feelings, goals, and choices as well as provide valuable emotional support. Counseling

may be undertaken on an individual basis for the person with MS or for a family member, a couple, or a family unit. Group counseling can be particularly helpful, as it provides an opportunity to discuss common problems and issues with others in similar circumstances. (See discussion on this subject in Chapter 13.) The interchange is maximized by the participation of a professional group leader as opposed to self-help or "rap" groups. Your physician, the local chapter of the National MS Society, or local mental health center can help define the services available in a particular community.

ONGOING PROBLEMS

Questions about interpersonal relationships persist as time goes by. One such problem involves "role expectations" or ways of behaving and reacting in situations that fit with self-image and the expectations of those around you. This includes attitudes, activities, patterns of decision-making, expressing feelings, and meeting needs of significant others. Role expectations exist in every social situation but are of greatest importance within the home and with those people with whom one is in daily or intimate contact. Some thought should be given to determine current role expectations and the ways that these might be threatened by the diagnosis of a chronic disease or by actual physical disability. A determined effort may be needed to minimize those changes that will have undesirable outcomes. Awareness of potential problem areas and pitfalls may be helpful in anticipating difficulties and bypassing disastrous outcomes.

Relationship with Parents

Look at current roles and relationships with family members such as parents. How frequent are visits and telephone contacts with them (if not living in the same household)? During times of particular stress, such as the appearance of new symptoms or a job change, an increase in contacts can be expected. However, a general pattern of calling more often and allowing more activities to be undertaken by parents unnecessarily should be a warning that dependency may be growing.

Given the earlier parent/child roles, it is easy for this to happen and more difficult to reverse than to prevent. It is important to be aware of the love and concern motivating parents to "do something" and to emphasize the importance of the MS person's need to maintain as much independence as possible when discussing the situation with them. Parents generally want to be helpful and appreciate honesty about how best to accomplish this. If circumstances require that more assistance be provided, relinquishing tasks or specific responsibilities to parents may be needed and greatly appreciated. Frank discussion along with accurate identification of tasks requiring assistance can facilitate the MS person's control over how help is distributed and utilized.

Parents of a young adult with MS who find themselves in the quandary of wanting to be helpful while not encouraging dependence may also find some structured reflection helpful. They may begin by considering the amount of current contact (phone calls, visits) versus that prior to diagnosis. Which of these changes reflect (a) a need for direct care because of progressive disability, (b) relief of some activities and/or responsibilities because of progressive disability, and (c) assumption of activities or responsibilities that might still be managed by the MS person? Unfortunately, certain activities may need to be relinquished by the individual, depending on the level of disability. However, the greatest favor is to assist the daughter or son to continue previous activities as much as possible. The desire to help can often be directed toward devising creative ways to make this happen: for example, suggest a telephone bill-paying service, use of a device such as the Amigo to increase mobility, the use of hand controls on the car, etc. Modifications will need to be individually designed according to abilities and limitations. In those rare situations where disability is extensive, parents may find themselves assuming increasing responsibility for care without much freedom for deciding the limits. Even in such severe circumstances, choices still exist: the choice to care for the MS individual without outside help, to seek outside help from public or private agencies, to delegate care to an appropriate facility such as a health-related facility (HRF) or nursing home (skilled nursing facility or SNF). Such decisions may be best for all concerned but are usually accepted better when made with consultation of a health professional such as the physician, nurse, or social worker. Parents are not able to assume responsibility for the well-being of their child forever, particularly as MS does not often decrease life expectancy, and long-term plans must be considered.

Guilt is a common response of parents whose child has MS, possibly because of earlier roles of parental responsibility. Realistically, parents and others have no control over precipitating the onset of MS. This knowledge may not diminish the pain of such feelings, however, and professional counseling might be indicated to help parents relieve these and other painful and confusing responses.

Not all parents experience the desire to be helpful as the primary reaction. Anger, depression, and rejection may be prolonged emotional responses. In these cases, the parent's life situation may make assuming responsibility for the MS person totally unrealistic or undesirable. As stated previously, feelings are neither "good" nor "bad" in a moral sense. The parent who has struggled for many years to achieve an independent life-style or retired people who at last are experiencing long-planned freedom are examples of parents who may very appropriately fear having a disabled son or daughter increasingly dependent on them. In most cases, additional physical and/or fiscal responsibility is not relegated to parents, as most people with MS do not become severely disabled. The fear and dread of this possibility, however, is very real. Acceptance of such responses by the parents themselves, the MS person, and others involved with the family can clear the way for an ongoing open and mutually supportive relationship.

Parent–child relationships are complicated in the best of circumstances, and MS only increases the confusion. It is important to remember that all involved are entitled to feel angry, depressed, and resentful. Awareness of the source of these feelings and open communication between family members help bring these painful feelings into proper perspective and increase the intimacy and support already present.

Relationship with Children

This discussion refers to preschool and school-age children, as these children are living at home and are directly affected by MS in the household. The MS parent and spouse with young or teenage children face many decisions about how to deal with MS within the family unit. Unfortunately, parents may underestimate their children and believe that denial will effectively cover up the problems of MS. These parents unwittingly communicate their worry, anxiety, and distress while trying to assure the child that everything is fine. The perceptive child may outwardly react to the verbal statements while harboring fearful fantasies. Deception about such a vital area as a parent's health implies that the truth is devastating or "unspeakable." The child may then exhibit acceptance because he or she has received the message that speaking openly about this topic is prohibited. The loneliness and fright the child conceals, however, may be acted out in other ways because such feelings are not easily contained. Academic difficulties, fights with classmates, truancy, withdrawal, and even delinquency can be emotional outlets for these painful feelings. These events certainly occur in the absence of MS but are more likely when the family has closed off the possibility of sharing problems openly.

The goal is not to tell children elaborate details of symptoms and potential complications. The kind of information communicated depends on the child's age, his or her ability to comprehend, and the questions asked. Appropriate articles can be given to teenagers if interest is expressed.

Advocating openness with children is not meant to imply that this will prevent or solve all potential problems surrounding the parent's MS. Should disability develop, the child's adjustment to living in a family with chronic illness can be especially difficult. Children will also be affected by the uncertainty and fluctuation of symptoms, as are the parent with MS and other close family members. The younger child's unsophisticated level of verbal communication and limited life experience occasionally create a situation best alleviated by professional counseling. A need for such counseling does not reflect inadequacies of the parents. Rather, it reflects the confusing and bewildering impact of chronic disease in the family superimposed on the normally difficult developmental tasks of growing up. Professionals who are trained in eliciting information from children are invaluable. Usually only several sessions will be needed to clarify problem areas and assist parents and child to choose effective ways of handling them.

Relationship with the Spouse

There is often a parallel between the MS person's response to chronic illness and the spouse's response. For example, the couple tends either to pursue the same patterns of socialization that existed prior to the illness or to isolate themselves from former social relationships. This dichotomy refers primarily to MS in which disability is apparent or activities are limited by easy fatigability. When isolation is chosen as the predominant pattern, it is usually a result of a reduction in the family's free time because of management of the impairment and, more significantly, of negative attitudes attributed to people outside the family. It appears that the preconception of people's reaction to physical limitation is more powerful than actual experiences. This suggests that the attitudes of the couple (more than the degree of disability) limit socialization with others. The couple need to examine their own earlier attitudes toward people with physical limitations and the resultant influence on current interpretation of other people's responses. It is also important to consider that people respond to behavior, so that the couple who convey discomfort and awkwardness elicit a similar response. Lacking awareness of this phenomenon, the couple may attribute all negative reactions to the disability. As stated earlier, such a simplified explanation is not intended to minimize the difficult adjustments that may be needed but to provide a basis for understanding and a direction for growth.

The couple's relationship with each other is also directly affected by the MS of one partner. Open communication is the basis for adjustment, assuming the preexistence of love and trust between the spouses. The stress of a chronic illness can heighten previous interpersonal conflicts, so that positive factors need to be emphasized. Both partners will experience feelings such as anger, despair, loneliness, and self-pity—all very appropriate to the current situation. If these feelings can be shared, the sense of aloneness can be reduced. An effort by each spouse to understand the other's feelings may not only strengthen the relationship but provide an atmosphere conducive to problem solving and defining mutual goals. Adjustments must be made by both partners, a process that may necessitate dealing with very strong emotions and allowing more separate "space" than before. For example, consider a couple who enjoyed playing tennis together and can no longer do so because of the limitations of one partner. Both are resentful, but the disability of one spouse need not be imposed on the other. The non-MS partner can continue this activity and may need encouragement to do so. The spouse with MS may become active in political groups that promote the rights of disabled individuals and also needs approval to do so. What may appear as distancing in such a relationship actually allows for more freedom to enjoy each other with little resentment. Spouses need to retain separate identities despite areas of dependence that may be necessitated by MS.

Individuality, interdependence, and mutual love and respect can be maintained despite the impact of MS and should be important components of all interactions between spouses. Hopefully, these feelings will also facilitate their socialization within the community. This, fortunately, is the outcome for most couples dealing with MS.

Potential Dependency Issues (Spouses)

Potential dependence within the couple may involve emotional, physical, and/or economic aspects. Emotional dependence occurs when the MS partner relies almost exclusively on his or her spouse for socialization, encouragement, and attention. Outside relationships may be unnecessarily relinquished, as well as participation in family decision making. Physical dependence includes reliance by the MS partner on his or her spouse for assistance with personal activities such as bathing, dressing, and housekeeping or household maintenance tasks. Economic dependence results from diminished or lost income by the MS partner, thereby increasing the need for financial support from the non-MS spouse.

As these transitions occur, the MS person may experience feelings of frustration and a loss or reduction of the sense of self-worth. The spouse is likely also to have some negative reactions, including resentment and fear of losing a separate identity. One phenomenon that couples have described illustrates the change in patterns of relating to each other: In certain circumstances the nondisabled spouse serves as a physical or even mechanical extension of the MS person. The healthy spouse becomes the "legs," "hands," a retrieval device, or a messenger for the MS spouse. It is not the actual performance of tasks that is at issue, as these can be requested and carried out within the context of loving and caring communication. The negative interaction involves depersonalization of the nondisabled spouse, wherein commands replace requests. For the MS partner this is probably an expression of intolerable frustration, but it needs to be discussed openly if increasing resentment by the non-MS partner is to be avoided.

Emotional dependence can be eased by continued socialization with friends, both as a couple and as individuals. As noted previously, socialization is more limited by the couple's attitudes than by physical impediments, so the initiative to continue a social life must come from the couple. The disabled person can maintain friendships by telephone when get-togethers are not feasible. Both partners have a responsibility to themselves and to each other to continue valued personal and mutual friendships. This is important for each partner's self-image and enjoyment of life as well as for the health of the couple's relationship.

Another factor in preventing dysfunctional emotional dependency of one spouse is cultivation of an environment in which interdependence and mutual respect may develop or continue. The need for understanding, love, and encouragement is basic for most people and can be shared and exchanged despite physical limitations.

Physical dependence may develop because of specific MS impairments from weakness or decreased energy or as the result of psychological or attitudinal factors. Psychological factors include depression, "putting off" efforts while waiting for a remission, or the partner's desire to make life easier by taking on tasks rather than watch his or her spouse struggle to learn adaptive skills. These and other responses are counterproductive and need to be dealt with if physical dependence is to be kept within the boundaries of necessity.

Special problems arise when role reversal is encountered. This entails one or both spouses assuming tasks or responsibilities previously within the other partner's domain. The man whose wife has physical limitations from MS may need to take on unfamiliar childcare and housekeeping activities. The woman whose spouse becomes disabled may be confronted with household repairs, financial management, and perhaps economic support. These examples reflect traditional roles in our society and do not apply to every couple. Difficulties cannot be avoided in such circumstances, but frustration can often be eased and resentment minimized. Attitudes about male–female roles need to be flexible, and tasks reassigned or "swapped" according to the family needs and the abilities of both spouses. The homemaker who must switch to wage earner will appreciate whatever help is possible in household management from the home-bound partner. Unnecessary dependence occurs when this help does not materialize and the MS spouse withdraws from all responsibilities. Even the severely disabled individual can perform such tasks as compiling grocery lists and calling in orders to local stores for home delivery (special telephone devices are available for the disabled, as well as operator-transmitted calls). Too often, effort is not expended by the disabled spouse to find creative ways of performing tasks or assuming new responsibilities. It is this apathy that can heighten interpersonal tension to the breaking point. Working together, at each partner's maximal level of functioning, helps maintain a positive and caring relationship.

Economic dependence resulting from decreased income and compounded by mounting medical expenses can be the source of severe interpersonal conflict. This corresponds with couples who do not have to deal with chronic illness, where financial problems are often the core of marital conflict. Some measures can be taken to reduce this high-risk problem area. The first and crucial step is to be sure that maximal health-care insurance is in effect for the MS partner and family. The increased cost of premiums for such coverage is worth the added expense. Policies should be checked to verify coverage in the following areas: outpatient medical visits and procedures, outpatient and hospital rehabilitation, general hospital care and extended hospitalization, psychotherapy, home-care services, medications, supplies, and equipment. Depletion of financial resources may be avoided by this precaution, as medical expenses in chronic illness may become astronomical.

Consideration should also be given to benefit programs such as disability available through work and/or state and federal programs. These resources may be tapped under certain circumstances, thereby preserving personal assets. Consultation with a trusted and knowledgeable lawyer or accountant may clarify measures that will ensure continued financial stability and family security (such as trust funds for the children or mortgage disability insurance plans).

Another important concept is continued employment when the MS spouse is a wage earner. Apart from valuable effects such as maintenance of self-esteem and work socialization, the continuing income is certainly an asset. Related vocational/occupational issues are addressed in Chapter 15.

SUMMARY

The unpredictable and sometimes progressive course of MS undoubtedly presents a variety of problems. However, the MS person and family can do a great deal to develop satisfactory patterns for coping with the ongoing stresses. Assistance from health professionals may give needed direction and support for strategies of adaptation. Armed with accurate information and professional guidance when needed, the MS individual and family can determine the most appropriate measures to achieve optimal function and quality of life.

15

Vocational Issues

Nancy J. Holland, Seymour R. Kaplan, and Harry L. Hall

One of every four persons with MS is working, and another is very interested in returning to employment. Despite medical, functional, and environmental problems sometimes associated with MS, many persons with MS are capable of performing appropriate employment during part or all of their working age. In fact, as the capacity to treat/manage secondary symptoms has improved, and as the other issues related to employment of persons with MS have become better understood, an increasing number of persons with MS have sought to obtain and retain employment.

The uncertainty with respect to future course of the disease in any individual is a difficulty. The multiplicity of symptoms in conjunction with fatigue often create special circumstances. The pattern of exacerbations and remissions sometimes requires work schedule modifications. Multiple sclerosis symptoms prevent employment for some persons, but for most persons with MS working depends primarily on:

1. Coping mechanisms and the capacity to manage one's own life.
2. Employment opportunities that maximize interests, skills, education, and experience and minimize the impact of functional limitations.
3. "Reasonable accommodations" if necessary.

For many people, positive feelings about themselves are at least partially related to job or career roles. The diagnosis of a chronic disease such as MS always threatens the individual's self-image but has a much greater impact when work activity is affected. Every effort

230   VOCATIONAL ISSUES

should be made to maintain the individual's confidence and prior level of function. The potential work dropout may be facing considerable physical limitations or responding to depression, anticipation of disability, or adoption of the sick role. Whether the cause is physical or emotional, the process requires interruption at this point. It is more difficult to resume employment status than to maintain it; regaining self-esteem presents a far greater obstacle than retaining it. Although unemployment may accrue financial benefits, it can have profound repercussions: the handicapped identity is assumed, expectations of career advancement are canceled, and dependence on the government for financial support is established.

It might be helpful at this point to differentiate among some commonly used terms that may seem interchangeable but which have subtle and significant differences. These definitions were prepared by the World Health Organization, and efforts are under way to promote them for international usage:

Impairment refers to the physical defect caused by MS lesions with resultant loss of normal bodily mechanical function.

Disablement refers to the consequences of impairment with a reduction in functional ability.

Handicap refers to the effects of impairment or disability on the person's interactions with others and the ability to keep a satisfactory place in the community.

To illustrate these definitions, consider a person with severe visual deficiency. The actual limitation in vision is an *impairment*. When the visual problem interferes with function, such as reading or writing checks, it becomes a *disability*. When this individual applies for a job as a taxi driver or engraver, the visual deficiency may be considered by others as a *handicap*.

According to this terminology, measures can be taken to prevent some impairments from being disabilities. In the case mentioned, eyeglasses or a magnifier might suffice. Likewise, some handicaps can be avoided. The visually impaired person might work as a consumer advocate or insurance agent, and the visual problem may not be regarded as a handicap.

These distinctions are not merely semantic exercises but are intended to convey a realistic perspective. The impairment, or physical limitation, is usually a factor over which the individual has little control. Some choices do exist, however, as to the extent that impairment becomes a disability or handicap. These choices are particularly evident in the area of vocational adaptation.

VOCATIONAL ASSESSMENT

Changes in physical status may necessitate a reassessment of abilities and limitations relative to work requirements. Because intellect is not usually impaired, skills can be redirected and utilized.

When a career change is not indicated, certain modifications may be helpful. Professional guidance and assistance with vocational problems are available through various agencies.

State agencies that offer rehabilitation services are sometimes called bureaus, offices, departments, or divisions of vocational rehabilitation. The program, often referred to as "VR," is mandated by law (The Rehabilitation Act). Agencies provide assistance to disabled persons who want to become employed or who need help to retain their jobs. Among the services are:

1. Evaluation of employment potential (vocational evaluation), including medical evaluation and occupational preference testing.
2. Counseling and guidance, including vocational and personal adjustment counseling.
3. Vocational and other job-training services, including work experience, training materials, and education.*
4. Financial maintenance during rehabilitation.*
5. Transportation related to rehabilitation services.*
6. Services to family members when such services aid the rehabilitation of the disabled person.
7. Technological aids and devices.*
8. Assistance in obtaining employment opportunities.
9. Occupational licenses, tools, and equipment.*
10. Postemployment follow-up services.

---

* Availability of this service may be based on economic need.

Individuals with vocational difficulties may apply to state vocational agencies themselves or be referred by a physician, other health practitioner, or a chapter of the National Multiple Sclerosis Society.

The current disabled population in the United States numbers about 30 million, of whom about 200,000 have MS. Of particular interest to the MS person are the 1977 and 1983 cooperative agreements between representatives of private and public sectors to increase and improve vocational services for the MS population. The involved agencies include:

1. Rehabilitation Services Administration (RSA, a federal agency with very substantial federal resources).
2. National Multiple Sclerosis Society (NMSS, a private voluntary organization that promotes and supports research and services related to MS).
3. Council of State Administrators of Vocational Rehabilitation (CSAVR, those state programs designed to help the disabled retain or regain productive employment).
4. The National Institute on Disability and Rehabilitation Research (NIDRR, formerly the National Institute of Handicapped Research).

The goals and objectives of these agreements have been pursued by agency actions that have improved the quantity and quality of services as well as the number of persons having success.

For those individuals who are seeking employment, the Rehabilitation Act of 1973 provides useful protection. This act requires that employers holding federal contracts for $2,500 or more take affirmative action to hire the disabled (Section 503), and it prohibits discrimination against disabled persons in all employment practices. This mandate encompasses approximately half of the businesses in America. The 1973 act also directs the employer to make "reasonable accommodations" for the handicapped employee (Section 504). This includes making facilities more accessible (such as restrooms, equipment, and work areas) by installing ramps and other adaptations.

Persons with multiple sclerosis who are eligible for government income and health care programs remain "medically" eligible unless symptoms improve significantly over an extended period of time. The law includes special provisions for "disabled" persons when they test their ability to work. Provisions for those who receive Social Security Disability Insurance (SSDI) include the following:

1. A "trial work" period of 9 months when income benefits continue to be paid regardless of earned income.
2. A 3-month adjustment period after successful trial work when income benefits are also paid.
3. An additional 15-month period after successful trial work when income benefits can be immediately restarted by notifying the Social Security Administration that work ("substantial gainful activity") has stopped.
4. A 5-year period after income benefits stop when a new "waiting period of 5 months" is not required.
5. For persons working part-time, a continuation of income benefits if monthly earnings do not exceed a limit ("substantial gainful activity" limit plus allowable "impairment-related work expenses").

Medicare benefits are obtained by persons eligible for SSDI after receiving income benefits for 2 years. Subsequent "waiting periods" have been eliminated by law. Medicare coverage is continued for 2 years after income benefits have ceased for disabled persons who have returned to employment. Thus, Medicare coverage usually continues for 3 years after the beginning of "trial work."

A slightly different but similar pattern of provisions (referred to as 1619a&b) is available to persons receiving Supplemental Security Income (SSI) and state Medicaid benefits. Provisions of private pensions and health care policies are widely divergent. Since many employer group health plans include a 6-month to 1-year "precondition clause," temporary continuation of existing health insurance is a consideration for those without continuing Medicare or Medicaid coverage.

VOCATIONAL REHABILITATION AGENCIES

Various agencies are concerned with providing social and vocational services for people with disability. Agencies vary from community to community, although those that are federally administered are fairly consistent. Eligibility is based on residence within the particular state and existence of a handicapping physical or psychological disability.

When the impairment includes a severe visual disability, a state agency for the blind and visually handicapped may be the appropriate state agency for vocational services. Requirements include visual acuity of 20/200 (with best correction in the better eye) or limited peripheral vision of 20° or less. These impairments are classified as "legal blindness," although some functional vision is often present.

PROJECTS WITH INDUSTRY

The Rehabilitation Services Administration is funding "Projects with Industry," which assists people with various types of disabilities to find satisfying jobs. One of these, the "Einstein Project," supports a program called "Job Raising" in collaboration with the National Multiple Sclerosis Society. The Development Team, Inc., based in Arlington, VA, together with the Medical Rehabilitation Research and Training Center for MS at the Albert Einstein College of Medicine in The Bronx, NY, are managing the federal project. A prominent national advisory structure of business persons is involved. Employment activities are handled locally by chapters of the National MS Society. The chapters run job readiness training groups, which address such issues as resume preparation, interview skills, stress management, and improved self-confidence. When a person is ready to enter the competitive job market, he or she is matched with a volunteer partner in a key position within the appropriate field. The volunteer and person with MS work together to explore potential employment positions, utilizing the skills and business contacts of the volunteer. This program is appropriate for persons who have job skills that may be applied with only "reasonable" accommodations or modifications needed by the employer to compensate for the MS person's handicap. More information about this program can be obtained from the National MS Society or the Development Team, Inc. The following questionnaire utilized by the Einstein Project might be a helpful guide for those MS persons who are not working but are thinking about pursuing employment:

This self-screening inventory has no right or wrong answers. It is a tool to help individuals consider whether job readiness training and employment are appropriate at this time. The inventory was developed by the "Einstein Project," a national Project with Industry, for use by potential job seekers in chapters of the National Multiple Sclerosis Society conducting a Job-Raising program.

1. Am I interested in working?
Is a job important: to satisfy my desire to do something purposeful? to my self-esteem? to be with other people? to meet my financial needs or aspirations?
yes ( )   no ( )   uncertain ( )

2. Can I afford to work?
Have I considered financial implications? benefit restrictions? insurance coverage issues? family needs? transportation expenses? and/or other factors which might dissuade me from taking a job? (This may require more details than you presently have. Get the facts; they are often different from commonly held prejudgments.)
yes ( )   no ( )   uncertain ( )

3. Can I work?
Am I able to work if I find the right job? Am I presently doing volunteer/community/home activities that are similar to some employment activities? Am I physically able to work? (If "uncertain," seek professional advice.)
yes ( )   no ( )   uncertain ( )

4. Do I have job qualifications?
Do I have previous work experience? education? volunteer experience? hobbies? and/or other skills marketable to employers?
yes ( )   no ( )   uncertain ( )

5. Can I develop realistic employment goals?
Do my job qualifications match the types of employment in which I have a real interest? Am I open to seriously considering career plans and income ranges that are consistent with my current capabilities?
yes ( )   no ( )   uncertain ( )

6. Can I improve my "readiness" to work?
Do I need help with: understanding work-related accommodations? stress management techniques? coping with MS symptoms on the job? vocational assessment? career planning? self-confidence? eligibility and benefit issues regarding social security, other disability insurances, or health insurance? use of other employment-related community resources?
yes ( )   no ( )   uncertain ( )

7. Can I improve my job-seeking skills?
Do I need help with: resume and cover letter preparation? researching potential employers? job search techniques? interviewing techniques? disclosing MS and asking for needed accommodations?
yes ( )   no ( )   uncertain ( )

8. Am I willing to involve others in my job search?

Am I willing to contact friends and others regarding job leads? Am I willing to accept: advice? assistance from a business person? mutual support from other job seekers? help from a community program? Am I willing to follow through with suggested contacts?
yes ( )   no ( )   uncertain ( )

9. Am I willing to commit to a formal program designed to help? Am I willing to: complete an eight-session Job Readiness Training program? meet with a vocational rehabilitation counselor? form a job-seeking partnership with a volunteer business leader? participate in a mutually supportive relationship with other job seekers?
yes ( )   no ( )   uncertain ( )

If most of your answers are affirmative, please contact the chapter staff to discuss your interest and learn more about Job Raising.

Which of the following employment-related options interest you? full-time employment ( ) part-time or flex-time employment ( ) transitional or trial work ( ) change to a more appropriate job ( ) retaining present job ( ) volunteer work that may lead to a job ( )

POSSIBLE ADAPTIVE MEASURES

There are many potential alterations the person with MS can consider in order to keep or secure a job. Choices depend on the individual's difficulties and needs, work environment and job description, imagination, and determination. The following are representative options for consideration as well as ideas to stimulate the development of other adaptive measures.

1. Fluctuating energy levels may be circumvented by work that is task-oriented rather than time-oriented, has intermittent or staggered work hours, or allows lunch-time naps; self-employment and homebound work on consignment are also possibilities.
2. Physical limitations may be overcome by shifting from a physically demanding job to a sedentary one. Consider transfer to a company where appropriate positions are available or architectural barriers are absent.
3. Commuting difficulties can be minimized by employment within a more geographically accessible area. A desirable locale might be one along a negotiable bus route or within a financially reasonable taxi zone. Private taxi companies may provide assistance

with appliances such as a walker or wheelchair for regular customers. Participation in a car pool is also a possibility.
4. Adaptive devices can compensate for some physical impairments. Some examples:
   a. Automobile hand controls when driving ability is affected by leg weakness or incoordination.
   b. Voice amplification devices when weak vocal projection is a problem.
   c. Optical aids to offset some visual impairments.
   d. Calculators, electric typewriters, and remote control units to compensate for upper extremity involvement.
   e. Assistance devices for ambulation, such as a cane or walker, to afford greater mobility and help prevent falls.
   f. Motorized "scooters," such as the Amigo and Portascoot, when mobility or easy fatigability is a problem.

In addition to hand controls, procurement of a "disabled driver's parking permit" increases access by automobile. Also, a citizen-band transmitter/receiver installed in the car can be utilized to summon assistance during an emergency. For the disabled driver, even a flat tire may produce a crisis situation if help is not nearby.

For those using public transportation, the cost can be reduced by the "Half-Fare Program for the Handicapped" available in most communities.

More ideas for adaptive measures to support occupational efforts directly or indirectly can be found in Chapter 9.

SUMMARY

Working provides an important source of self-esteem and financial independence for many people, including those with MS. Maintenance of employment is more easily achieved than reemployment, and so every effort should be made to continue work activities with whatever modifications are needed. Assistance is often available for those who desire to return to work. People with MS seeking to obtain/retain employment can hope to find many possibilities available to them.

Multiple Sclerosis: A Guide for Patients and Their Families, Second Edition, edited by L. C. Scheinberg and N. J. Holland. Raven Press © 1987.

16

What About New Treatments?

Robert J. Slater and Labe C. Scheinberg

There are many reasons why the person with MS is frequently confused, frustrated, and even cynical regarding treatments and claims for ending progression or bringing about remission of the disease. It is not yet possible to produce agents that will prevent the disease or alter its natural course over any long period. When remissions occur, they may be coincidental to interventions, although some drugs may shorten an exacerbation. Once a symptom or sign has become chronic, there is little likelihood that any intervention will reverse the patient's condition to that prior to the onset or worsening.

Two factors play a role in the failure of restoration of function: myelin in the central nervous system of man does not regenerate, and once a chronic scar has formed at the site of myelin breakdown, the nerve impulse transmission is impaired, and the scar is permanent. It is believed that remissions are a result of subsidence of the acute inflammation and not the regrowth of myelin.

Therapy in multiple sclerosis is divided into (a) prevention of its onset—not currently feasible; (b) halting the progression of the disease or "cure"—the area wherein most clinical trials are under way; (c) restoration to the predisease status—not currently feasible because of the factors just mentioned; and (d) treatment of certain specific symptoms such as spasticity or bladder dysfunction.

It is currently held by most scientists that multiple sclerosis is a result of an autoimmune disorder, perhaps coupled with a viral infection. As with other chronic illnesses perhaps caused by autoimmune reactions (for instance, rheumatoid arthritis, lupus erythematosus, and myasthenia gravis), only a breakthrough in research will focus on what is wrong and what specific treatment is necessary. It is well to remember that such breakthroughs have been made in other illnesses, for example, vaccines to prevent polio and measles, antibiotics for many bacterial infections, insulin to control diabetes, and L-DOPA to control parkinsonism. In each of these examples, either a causative agent or a specific physiological defect was identified. Multiple sclerosis has other features that make the solution elusive. The course of the disease is unpredictable, and although at certain times the patient may appear to be improving, the number of lesions in the brain, shown by such tests as magnetic resonance imaging or evoked responses, may be increasing. The course of the disease usually occurs over many decades with unpredictable attacks and remissions. Placebo effects are apparent in many so-called cures, and other factors such as emotions, fatigue, concurrent infections, and environment play a major role in how the patient feels when evaluated.

At this time, physicians are excited about how much new information is arising from research, and though uneven, it is felt that progress is being made. Many clinical trials in multiple sclerosis have given false hope even when performed by competent, well-intentioned investigators, and many reported successes by those less experienced in the vagaries of the disease and in clinical research have given false hope and added to the confusion that exists. Frequently, the media report a new development in research that is immediately interpreted as relevant by overenthusiastic researchers and science reporters for a variety of reasons. The patients and their families and friends seize on these reports only to have their hopes dashed with the passage of time.

FACTORS INFLUENCING THE PATIENT'S RESPONSE

In order to judge what to do until we find a specific treatment, a number of factors must be considered. First, there is the problem of interpreting the natural clinical course of exacerbations and remissions. Some individuals may have a few attacks at onset, with complete clearing, and be symptom-free for the remainder of their lives. Others may relentlessly progress with increasing disability and experience no remissions. And finally, a large proportion fall somewhere in between these two extremes. The attacks are entirely unpredictable in their frequency, nature, and severity; each patient is unique. For example, if one patient has started a new diet or drug treatment, improvement may occur coincidentally, and one does not know if this was a spontaneous remission or a result of the diet or drug. It is also important to know when the treatment was begun in relation to the timing of the disease. Early in the disease, about three-quarters of the patients will experience some remission regardless of the treatment or even if none was administered. Also, if treatment is initiated when the course has already begun to improve, a rapid remission may occur and be interpreted as a result of the new therapy. Because of the unpredictable timing and severity of MS bouts from one person to the next and one attack to the next in the same patient, it is usually impossible to determine benefits of any treatment for many years.

One way to overcome this problem is to use a large number of patients and to divide these randomly into two groups: the experimental group receiving therapy and the placebo group who get an inactive substance resembling the active agent. Neither the patient nor the physician is aware of who is in each group. This is the design for a randomized, double-blind clinical trial. In order to obtain sufficient numbers to complete the study in a reasonable period of time, the studies are often done in many centers. Although this may eliminate the bias of a particular center, it introduces the problem of variation from one examiner or group of examiners to another. Moreover, it is often difficult to blind either the physician or the patient. Every active ingredient has some side effect, however subtle, and the physician or patient is often aware to which group the patient has been randomized. Additionally, patients will occasionally deny side effects in order to remain in the treatment group or even give the proper response to gain entry into a study. It has been readily admitted that entry criteria for popular clinical trials form a frequent topic in patient support groups. When cases are solicited by advertising on television or in the newspaper, one can be assured that many subjects will be sophisticated and give the appropriate responses to be selected. For best results, the patients should be known to the investigators for several years prior to entry so that the actual course is known and has been documented.

Another factor in understanding how the body responds in multiple sclerosis is the ability for self-healing (spontaneous remission). This seems to be augmented at times by belief that a particular treatment will help. This is called the placebo response. Because of the strong influence of our personality and behavior on how our bodies respond, the placebo response can mimic a positive response to treatment in over half the patients. Although objective changes may not occur, the patient may be motivated to exert more effort and perform better during the examination.

The placebo reponse is clearly a part of the doctor–patient relationship and is augmented when these experiences of faith and hope are shared by others in a group. Having some form of faith and optimism is a very important part of maintaining a positive and hopeful outlook on life. The behavioral responses set in motion are increasingly understood to be associated with stress reduction. Norman Cousins noted the powerful effect of faith in the partnership with his physician and how self-determination to reduce worry and stress by positive thinking resulted in a profound healing effect. Although this may be noted in the early acute phases, one should not depend on this to produce reversal of findings that have been present for more than a year or so.

Understanding that stress may be harmful, leading to damage of various parts of the body, is an important incentive to find ways to reduce stress on a day-to-day basis and perhaps minimize the effects of progression or attacks.

Research has indicated that behavioral variations that result from stress are probably mediated by hormones produced in the brain that regulate responses in the nervous system, cardiovascular system, gastrointestinal system, genitourinary system, etc. The implications of these normal behavioral responses, which affect us all, are important in assessing both the patients' and physicians' approach to unproven therapies. The positive placebo effect is so important in MS therapy that it might be stated that the real cure for multiple sclerosis is one that halts attacks or progression and causes improvement even if neither the physician nor the patient believes in it.

It is understandable that patients are usually anxious about their future and sometimes desperate. There are instances when patients have become involved in more than one clinical trial at the same time or have taken other treatments while engaged in a clinical trial without informing their physician. One patient typified this when she was involved in a trial of one agent and unwittingly said to one of the naive authors (L.C.S.), who was administering steroids for an acute attack, "Do you think that I should tell Dr. X (the principal investigator of the trial in which she was involved) that I am taking hyperbaric oxygen treatments from Dr. Y?" It is little wonder that one has difficulty in evaluating the results of therapy in MS.

TYPES OF CLINICAL TRIALS

Clinical trials are divided into preliminary, pilot, and full clinical trials. In the preliminary trial, one attempts to establish dosage, study toxicity, and obtain a lead to the possible efficacy of a new treatment. In this type of study, the patient usually serves as his own control (the patient's condition pretherapy is compared with his status following therapy). The aim of the pilot study is to learn if a treatment that looked good in the preliminary trial still looks good when tested under more rigorously controlled conditions. These are usually performed in a single institution and in a carefully selected group of patients. If one or more pilot studies indicate a clinically significant beneficial effect without serious side effects, then one would proceed to a full clinical trial. A full clinical trial is carried out to determine whether the results seen in the pilot study are real and have general applicability. This involves using concurrent controls (patients with a similar disease course who are not receiving the experimental therapy), randomization, and double-blinding.

All clinical trials require the approval of the institutional review board (hospital or medical school usually) and signing of informed consent by the patient. There should be adequate staff to have both a blinded examiner and an unblinded physician to monitor the laboratory tests and change dosages or stop treatment if necessary. Before any agent is tested, approval from the Food and Drug Administration is required. This agency's final approval must be obtained prior to the

TABLE 1. *New treatments undergoing clinical trials*

Rationale	Status
Antiinflammatory	
ACTH (corticotropin)	Further trials under way; widely employed for acute attacks only
Steroids (prednisone and others; intraspinal, oral, high-dose i.v.)	Further trials under way; widely employed for acute attacks only
Colchicine	New pilot trials under way; no data published as yet
Immune system	
Azathioprine (Imuran)	Further trials under way; pilot trials encouraging
Cyclophosphamide (Cytoxan)	Further trials under way; pilot trials encouraging
Cyclosporin	Trials under way; preliminary results not available
Monoclonal antibodies	Further trials under way; preliminary results not encouraging
Plasmapheresis	Further trials under way; preliminary results are controversial
Lymphocytapheresis	Further trials under way; preliminary results are controversial
Total lymphoid irradiation	Further trials under way; preliminary results have not been confirmed
Thymosin	Further trials under way; preliminary results not available
Copolymer I	Further trials under way; preliminary results available only for exacerbations, where it seemed to be encouraging
Transfer factor	Further trials under way; preliminary results not encouraging
Antiinfective	
Human immunoglobulin	Further trials under way; preliminary results not encouraging
Interferon (systemic, intraspinal, and intrabrain injection)	Further trials under way; preliminary results not encouraging; results are confused because there are a "variety of interferons"
Hyperimmune bovine colostrum	Very controversial and not accepted by most of medical profession
Miscellaneous empirical	
Hyperbaric oxygen	Numerous trials have shown its ineffectiveness
Dorsal column stimulation	Trials allegedly under way, but the value is very dubious, and it is not an accepted procedure for treatment of MS
Cobra venom	FDA has not approved for clinical trial because of contamination of serum with other reptile venoms

agent being released for general prescribing. This process requires a long period of time (usually 5 or more years) and vast sums of money. It is essential, nonetheless, to protect the public from harmful or even fatal treatments. The past history of drugs such as thalidomide are stark reminders of the necessity of these safeguards.

The therapies that are intended to shorten attacks, prevent attacks, slow or halt progression, and reverse the impairment are usually divided into (a) rational treatments (based on some generally accepted theory as to the cause of the disease) and (b) empirical treatments for which claims have been made and there is no known scientific basis. Though it may be an error to reject empirical treatments based on anecdotes, one cannot accept these without objective examination and well-controlled clinical trials.

The therapies of current interest that affect the course and outcome of the disease can be divided into antiinflammatory, immunosuppressive, immune modulators, and antiinfective agents. These are reviewed briefly, as are some of the popular empirical treatments, in Table 1.

SUMMARY

In summary, all the treatments listed in Table 1 are unproven and vary from rational to empirical and highly controversial. Some are expensive and not reimbursable by insurance carriers. Others are given in approved clinical trials and require no financial expenditure by the patient. Some of the treatments carry a significant risk, e.g., dorsal column stimulation or intracerebral injections; others, e.g., cyclophosphamide and cyclosporin, have an unknown long-term risk and must be carefully monitored.

Although the burgeoning interest in clinical therapeutic trials is encouraging, the investigations vary greatly in the underlying rationale, quality of study design, and risk for the patient. Patients and concerned others should clearly understand and weigh costs, potential risks, and benefits before entering a clinical trial or embarking on an unproven treatment.

17

Available Services

Diann Geronemus

Care for MS patients is complex and presents ongoing problems for the patient, family, health care providers, and community. Needs for care are unpredictable and vary greatly, given the differing presentations, symptoms, and levels of disability found in MS. The illness itself poses difficult diagnostic and management dilemmas. Some MS problems are common to other chronic disabilities as well.

Regardless of the severity of the physical and psychological impairment, some type of care is required in the following areas: (a) pharmacologic intervention; (b) medical and vocational rehabilitation; (c) bladder and bowel therapy; (d) counseling for psychological and sexual adaptation; (e) modification of the home and work environment; (f) special adaptations for transportation, recreation, and other activities of daily living; and (g) advice on economic management. Ideally, the system of human services within which care is given is responsive to the unique problems confronting MS patients and families as well as those problems MS persons share with other persons suffering from chronic illnesses.

Previous chapters have discussed care for MS patients in the areas of pharmacologic intervention; treatment with physical measures, including occupational therapy and activities of daily living; social and vocational adaptations; nursing care; bowel and bladder management; and psychological and sexual adjustments. Here these subjects are discussed insofar as they relate to a broad framework of continuing comprehensive care for MS patients and their families and to some specific services and programs currently available under governmental and voluntary auspices.

PROVISION OF MEDICAL AND SOCIAL CARE

Short- and long-term management in MS comprises many interrelated medical and social problems. Management involves two types of professional organization: the medical model and the helping model. In the medical model the emphasis is on diagnosis and management, with care generally being rendered in a structured setting such as a hospital, clinic, or office. This type of care lends itself more readily to acute-phase, episodic problem solving. In the helping model there is an emphasis on "wellness," on helping the patient develop problem-solving techniques, and on establishing links to community-based services in order to assemble necessary psychosocial and rehabilitative services. It is within this framework that more emphasis is optimally placed on the needs of chronically ill persons and on the provision of long-term social supports for this population.

It is commonplace to hear of situations in which patients and families living with MS have been poorly handled, misdiagnosed, or, more basically, misunderstood. Unfortunately, unresponsiveness in short-term management may lead to unnecessary obstacles in the need for continuing adaptations and dynamic management in the course of a chronic illness such as MS. Barriers to effective care can occur in the medical, psychosocial, or rehabilitation spheres. For example, poor early psychological and social adaptations to changing roles and work capabilities may set up barriers to long-term patient and family adjustments, just as inadequate early evaluation of bowel and bladder symptoms can lead to embarrassing and at times life-threatening chronic medical problems.

Some basic problems have been identified that underlie the provision of services to MS patients and families. Some of these problems are inherent in the disease process itself, and others relate to the system within which needs arise and human services are developed to meet patient needs. These problems include (a) the long-term, protracted nature of the medical and psychosocial needs, (b) unpredictability in the clinical course and severity of the disease, (c) fragmentation under different sponsorship and location of the mix of human services available to meet needs and the wide variation of services from one community to another, (d) a lack of coherence or coordination among those fragmented services, (e) difficulty experienced by many patients in obtaining access to services, and (f) economic instability resulting from uncertain employment and income in addition to the unpredictable costs of medical and social services.

MATCHING SERVICE TO NEED

At this point it is useful to examine a model of care that matches human services to patients' needs. Any such model must take into account existing patterns of federal–state reimbursements for relevant services, the political realities of evolving institutions and laws, the values of the society in which the system exists, and the knowledge and attitudes of individuals who will influence the disabled person and family directly or indirectly. Coordination of services is the goal of such an organizational model. A conceptual framework consisting of a three-sided spectrum of resources can provide an optimal mix of services.

Governmental service departments (health, welfare, rehabilitation, etc.) are represented on one side. Community, private, and public service institutions and agencies are represented on the second side; and volunteer citizens comprise the third component. Some of this third sector operates under tax-exempt status as fund-raising agencies to provide specific services, and other volunteers function as agents of good will. Certain constraints are inherent in the development and implementation of services as a result of governmental regulations. In any case, close coordination and communication within the system are essential to generate optimal services.

THE TEAM APPROACH

Within the three-sided system of services described, it is necessary to bring together a variety of professionals and lay persons who possess the knowledge and capabilities for dealing with the range of problems presented by MS patients and families. This confluence of professionals is consistent with the "team approach" to patient management. The team has increasingly been found to be effective in the provision of care to populations with long-term needs such as those found in MS. The team approach involves the physician and professionals in such disciplines as nursing, social work, clinical psychology, occupational, speech, and physical therapy, vocational rehabilitation counseling, and the clergy. The team approach can be utilized with many types of medical and psychological problems and is practiced in varied settings. The composition of the team varies depending on two factors: the setting and the patients' needs. Team efforts are directed toward providing (a) openness of communication on behalf of the patients, (b) continuity of care, (c) a multitude of available services, (d) a stable knowledge base, (e) ongoing education about the illness and related problems, and (f) psychological as well as physical support systems.

The team can provide enormous support for the MS patient and family, beginning with the earliest symptoms, to the disclosure of a diagnosis, through the minor and major crises posed by the progression of the illness. Whenever financially and physically feasible, some combination of professionals is brought together as a team.

PROGRAMS AND SERVICES FOR THE DISABLED

Certain types of general information about programs and services are available as part of the coordinated care ideally provided by this team. This information forms an essential knowledge base for MS patients and families regardless of the type of symptomatology, the level of disability, and the system of care. A look at this informational base begins with a discussion of governmentally mandated programs for the disabled. We then consider treatment modalities for varying levels of disability in MS and finally look at services available in local communities that provide the necessary care and treatment.

Governmental Programs for the Disabled

Governmental benefits for the disabled are established by law and are subject to change. This is equally true for federal programs such as Medicare and Social Security and for federal–state programs such as Medicaid. Additionally, federal–state programs are subject to signficiant variations among the states. It is helpful, however, to discuss some of the more general and stable features of these programs as they are relevant to persons with MS. Under the Social Security laws there are two separate cash benefit programs for the disabled: Social Security Disability Insurance (SSDI) and Supplemental Security Income (SSI). There are also two programs of medical assistance: Medicare and Medicaid. Eligibility criteria for these programs vary and are directly or indirectly based on meeting (a) the programs' mandated definition of disability and (b) the mandated financial requirements.

Definition of Disability

To be considered disabled under the social security law, a person must have a physical or mental condition that prevents him from engaging in any substantial gainful activity (SGA) that exists in the national economy and is expected to last (or has lasted) for at least 12 continuous months. Inability to do your regular work does not constitute disability. One must be prepared to show that he or she is unable to engage in any other type of gainful employment in order to be considered. For example, if the patient previously worked as a salesclerk but medical evidence indicates that he is capable of light sedentary work (office work) and possesses appropriate skills, it is quite likely that the claim will be denied.

The Social Security Administration maintains a medical listing of impairments for each disability category. The medical criteria have been broadened since the first edition of this book. In MS this means that one must have (a) significant and persistent disorganization of motor functions in two extremities resulting in sustained disturbance of gross and dextrous movements or of gait and station; (b) very significant visual impairment or mental impairment; or (c) significant, reproducible fatigue of motor function with substantial muscle weakness on repetitive activity, demonstrated on physical examination, resulting from neurological dysfunction in areas of the central nervous system known to be pathologically involved by the MS process. Additional criteria since 1984 are evaluation of pain and consideration of the effects of multiple impairments. A combination of medical and vocational problems that make it extremely difficult to work may also meet the criteria. Given the great variability and unpredictability found in MS, it is the severity of the condition that must be documented.

The length of time and difficulty in making a diagnosis in MS pose a unique problem in disability determinations. Determining the date on which disability began can be crucial in SSDI cases because of the length of time involved in making the diagnosis of MS, during which MS patient's eligibility may have lapsed. Thus, it may be critical to convince the Social Security Administration that a patient actually had MS many years before a definite diagnosis was given and that the symptoms were severe enough to cause disability at the time the patient was still insured.

A detailed report is essential to any disability claim. Good and sufficient medical evidence will show the severity of the condition as well as the extent to which it prevents the patient from undertaking substantial gainful employment. Inadequate information at the outset may necessitate a laborious appeal procedure and, at times, the involvement of legal counsel. It is important to note that legally a substantially documented subjective symptom based on a verifiable medical condition such as MS may be grounds for disability. Such documentation may come from professionals or friends who have known the patient over a long period of time. This must be taken into consideration by the Social Security Administration even at the level of a hearing.

Cash Benefit Programs: SSDI

SSDI benefits are based on the patient's work history. For workers qualifying prior to July 1980, one must have worked 20 out of the previous 40 quarters (3-month periods) before becoming disabled, essentially 5 of the previous 10 years. For workers entitled to benefits July 1980 or later, there is a more complicated, graduated scale depending on the worker's age. This work requirement poses an obstacle to eligibility in MS with its greater number of female patients, as it excludes housewives who have been out of the competitive labor market for varying lengths of time. Once disability has been established, there is a 5-month waiting period until payments begin. In certain cases, retroactive payments up to 12 months may be applicable.

SSI

SSI is a public assistance benefit based on financial need rather than work history. One must meet maximum income and resource (savings, tangible assets) levels in order to qualify, as well as the disability requirements. SSDI benefits and the income of a nondisabled spouse are considered in the determination of SSI eligibility. How marital status affects income eligibility for SSI is a complicated issue and sometimes requires legal advice. States have the option of supplementing federal payments to SSI beneficiaries so that income criteria for this program vary from state to state. In certain cases where one is pursuing a vocational goal approved by the Social Security Administration and the state vocational rehabilitation agency, one may still be eligible for SSI under the self-support plan, even though income exceeds normal eligibility criteria. In such cases the cost of certain impairment-related items and services (transportation, equipment) needed in the pursuit of the vocational goal can be deducted from income and resources.

Medical Assistance Programs: Medicare

Medicare is a federally funded medical insurance program. A disabled person becomes entitled to Medicare after receiving SSDI benefits for 2 years (24 months). For disabled persons under the age of 65, this is the only means to eligibility for Medicare. The program has two parts: hospital insurance (part A) and medical insurance (part B). The former can help pay for medically necessary inpatient hospital care. Under certain circumstances it also covers inpatient care in a skilled nursing facility and care in the home by an approved home health agency. Medicare medical insurance can help pay for medically necessary doctors' services, outpatient hospital, physical therapy, and speech pathology services, and some medical services, supplies, and necessary home health services not covered by the hospital insurance part of Medicare. Medicare coverage does not pay the full cost of covered services.

Medicaid

Medicaid is a federal–state medical assistance program based on financial need. Financial eligibility requirements and services provided under the program vary from state to state. In some states Medicaid and SSI eligibility are the same, and one becomes eligible for both programs simultaneously.

Some states have a surplus (excess) income program. This allows the person with an income greater than that for Medicaid eligibility, but who meets all other requirements, to obtain Medicaid coverage by spending the "excess income" on medical expenses. Medicaid will then pay for medical expenses incurred. Medicaid is not a substitute for national health insurance and does not allow a middle-income family to keep its income and still be eligible for the program. In some states there is also a catastrophic health insurance provision.

Home Health Services

Different types of home health services are provided under the Medicare and Medicaid programs. Under the written plan of treatment of a physician, home health care services are provided under the Medicare program when the patient is homebound and requires intermittent skilled nursing, physical therapy, or speech therapy services. These include the insertion and sterile irrigation of catheters, application of dressings involving prescription medication and aseptic techniques, giving of injections, or performing physical therapy exercises. Personal care services can be provided by a home health aide for patients who require skilled nursing services. Medicare home health services do not provide what is considered custodial care (for example, feeding, bathing, transferring from bed to wheelchair). However, some of these needs may be met so long as a skilled nursing need is evident. There is no limit to the total number of home health care visits as long as the basic criteria are met. Medicare does not provide any home health services in what the program interprets as "chronic illness."

Medicaid home health care services vary widely from state to state. In some states the services and eligibility are similar to those of Medicare. In other states, provisions are broader and include some custodial care, housekeeper services for help with household chores, and homemaker services for help with shopping and preparing meals. The length of time that these services can be provided varies considerably from state to state.

Work Incentives

After successfully obtaining benefits under the cash benefit and medical assistance programs outlined, it is difficult to contemplate a return to work and subsequent loss of such benefits. Recent changes in the law are more supportive of a recipient's attempt to return to the work force while protecting his or her benefits. The law allows disabled persons to test their ability to work for a 9-month trial period and subsequent 3-month adjustment period while benefits continue. Some changes added by the 1980 Social Security Amendments include automatic reentitlement to benefits within 12 months if one again becomes unable to work after SSDI or SSI payments stop, continuation of Medicare benefits for 3 years after SSDI benefits cease because of a return to substantial gainful employment, reentitlement to Medicare immediately if a worker starts receiving SSDI benefits again within 5 years after they end and was previously entitled to Medicare, and allowing SSI recipients to return to work while continuing to receive Medicaid and social services necessary to maintain the work and cash benefits on a gradually decreasing scale.

Social Security laws are under continual review and revision. One can keep up with changes in the Social Security law by contacting the Social Security Administration and by contacting local legal services. Pamphlets discussing the various programs are available through the local Social Security office (Appendix A).

Care in the Voluntary Sector

Returning to our three-sided system of services, we now consider the care provided in the other two sectors—the community caregivers and citizens' groupings. Here, too, the types and extent of services available vary greatly from area to area and are based on perceived need, available physical and financial resources, the allocation of such resources, and the communication and collaboration between and among the populations in need and the persons and organizations providing services.

Services are based on a person's illness stage. The need for help varies according to the disability and must be responsive to the problems of (a) newly diagnosed patients and their families, (b) minimally to moderately disabled patients and their families, and (c) severely disabled patients and their families or caregivers. Certain needs and the services to meet them are common to all three levels. A natural movement in treatment approaches and service needs exists from one level to another. Specific goals and tasks of the service giver vary, as do the needs of the patient and family at any given level. It is important to note that in planning and providing any services there is a consideration of the total patient–family situation. It takes into account day-to-day needs, role relationships, values, perceptions of the consequences of the illness, vocational status, and family support systems.

Patients and families should find out about the services and resources available as early as possible. One might ask why such information should be obtained when there is no apparent problem as yet. We advocate getting complete information as early as possible in order to meet most expediently the long-term comprehensive need of MS persons and families. Knowledge about counseling programs, economic resources, equipment, and home care services can be readily accepted, less threatening, and less anxiety provoking if it is part of a total system of care. The knowledge can be integrated into long-term planning and problem solving with the goal of preventing crises or, at least, mitigating the effects of illness-related crisis situations. This becomes an educational process similar to the education about side effects of medication, bladder management, and skin care discussed in earlier chapters.

What do care and services mean for the MS patient and family? In broad groupings, these may include a range of counseling services, training programs, concrete services, and educational programs.

Counseling services include individual, group, couple, and family therapy; sexual counseling; and crisis intervention. In some areas specialized counseling services are available through MS clinical centers, MS chapter-supported programs, and neurology departments in medical centers. Such programs would be oriented to the specialized needs of the MS population and would involve various members of the professional team discussed earlier in this chapter. Group counseling would include professionally led groups and self-help groups organized and led by MS patients and families. Various types of therapy are also available through community-based family service and mental health agencies; the outpatient departments of hospitals and clinics; and private practitioners—physicians, clinical psychologists, social workers, marriage and family counselors, and the clergy.

Though it is not always the primary reason for entering therapy, MS will always have some impact on the treatment goals of therapy and the means taken to achieve them. At times, in the course of any of the forms of counseling mentioned, information regarding the illness, specific symptoms, and management may be shared (with the patient's permission) by the person providing the primary medical care and the therapist. This enhances understanding of the effects of the illness on adjustment in other areas, increases communication, and maximizes coordination of care for the MS patient and family.

Training programs are generally made available through the local offices of the state vocational rehabilitation agencies (OVR or DVR). Though not in the voluntary sector, they should be mentioned at this point. Vocational rehabilitation services may be available even if a person does not meet the requirements for disability benefits. These may include one or more of the following: counseling and guidance to discuss problems and interests in order to work out a rehabilitation program that may lead to achieving self-support; the provision of medical, surgical, or hospital services to reduce or remove disability; physical aids such as artificial limbs, braces, eyeglasses; job training in a vocational school, college, or rehabilitation facility; and job placement and follow-up.

Increasing numbers of MS patients throughout the country have become involved in state vocational rehabilitation programs since 1978 as a result of a joint agreement entered into by the National Multiple Sclerosis Society, the Rehabilitation Services Administration, and the Council of State Administrators of Vocational Rehabilitation. The purposes of the agreement were to work toward more effective coordination of these agencies' resources in order to increase education, promote early identification and referral of persons in need of rehabilitation, improve service techniques to MS persons, and increase the number of MS persons having gainful employment. A new agreement signed in 1983 adds the resources of the National Institute on Disability and Rehabilitation Research and continues and expands the stated purposes. Progress has been made in this area, though specific program activity varies from state to state. Some hospitals and rehabilitation centers offer limited vocational training, usually in a sheltered workshop setting, and in some areas voluntary agencies offer limited work opportunities and training.

Concrete services might include the provision of equipment, such as canes, walkers, wheelchairs, and Hoyer lifts. These may be obtained through the equipment loan programs of the local MS Society chapters. Some churches and fraternal organizations such as the Rotary, Elks, and Kiwanis may also have equipment available.

Homemaker and housekeeping services, transportation, and modifications to make a home accessible and barrier-free may be available through local community agencies and volunteer programs. Information about specialized services, such as hand controls and dwelling modifications, is available through rehabilitation centers and departments of physical and rehabilitation medicine in medical centers.

Talking books constitute another resource now more readily available to MS persons who have blurred or double vision, suffer from extreme weakness or excessive fatigue, are unable to hold a book or turn pages, or have other physical limitations that render them unable to read standard printed books. The limiting condition must be certified by a professional such as a physician, social worker, rehabilitation counselor, nurse, or therapist. Local public libraries and local chapters of the MS Society as well as the Division for the Blind and Physically Handicapped in the Library of Congress can supply more detailed information and application forms.

Education about MS—its symptoms, management, and the physical and emotional problems of daily living—is of considerable importance and should not be neglected in a chapter on care for the MS patient and family. Informal education must be considered a major resource. This involves actively soliciting information during medical visits, particularly where MS care is provided by a team with multiple professional disciplines represented. Literature about MS, problems of living with the illness, and some available services and resources are available through the National Multiple Sclerosis Society and its chapters. More formal educational programs for MS persons, families, and professionals are being developed by local MS chapters themselves and in conjunction with professional organizations such as medical societies and nursing associations.

It is important to note that all of the resources discussed in this section, even some of the governmental programs, vary considerably from area to area. Eligibility for programs and services is a major consideration, being based on financial as well as physical factors, and must be investigated on an individual case basis. Where questions exist as to the availability of services in a given area, there are some basic sources of information that can be helpful. These include the local MS Society chapters, which maintain a community resource file as part of their basic programs, community councils, community resource directories, hospital social service departments, and professional associations such as the local medical societies.

A chapter in a book such as this one seeks to apply theoretical formulations to the realities of seeking and providing care. With the knowledge base presented, one should be better prepared to obtain available resources in one's localities.

APPENDIX A: SOCIAL SECURITY ADMINISTRATION PAMPHLETS FOR THE DISABLED

A Brief Explanation of Medicare, HCFA, SSA Publication No. 05–10043.

A Guide to Supplemental Security Income, SSA, SSA Publication No. 05–11015.

A Message From Social Security: Why a Special Medical Examination Is Needed for Your Disability Claim. HHS Publication No. (SSA) 05–10087.

A Woman's Guide to Social Security. HHS Publication No. (SSA) 05–10127.

If You Become Disabled. HHS Publication No. (SSA) 05–10029.

Right to Appeal Supplemental Security Income. HHS Publication No. (SSA) 05–10281.

Your Medicare Handbook. HHS Publication No. (SSA) 05–10050.

Your Social Security. HHS Publication No. (SSA) 05–10035.

Your Social Security Rights and Responsibilities: Disability Benefits. HHS Publication No. (SSA) 05–10153.

SSI for Aged, Disabled, and Blind People. HHS Publication No. 05–11000.

What You Have to Know About SSI. HHS Publication No. (SSA) 05–11011.

A Special Message About SSI. HHS Publication No. (SSA) 05–11069.

Reporting Changes That Affect Your SSI Checks. HHS Publication No. (SSA) 05–11053.

How You Earn Social Security Credits. HHS Publication No. (SSA) 05–10072.

Social Security and Your Right to Representation. HHS Publication No. (SSA) 05–10075.

Your Right to Question the Decision Made on Your Social Security Claim. HHS Publication No. (SSA) 05–10058.

Your Disability Claim. HHS Publication No. (SSA) 05–10052.

Improvements in the Social Security Disability Program. HHS Publication No. (SSA) 05–10375.

Subject Index

Subject Index

Abdominal muscle, strengthening, 97
Acetaminophen, for body temperature elevation, 133
ACTH, 54,57,244
  dosage, 58
  side effects, 58–59
Acute myelitis syndrome, 44
Adrenocorticotropic hormone, see ACTH
Amantidine, 61
Amigo cart, 185
4-Aminopyridine, 65
Amitriptyline, 60,134
  dosage, 61
  indications for, 61
  side effects, 61
Anticholinergic agents
  glaucoma and, 157
  side effects, 62,157
Anticipation of disability, 79
  reinforcement, 79
Antivert, see Meclazine hydrochloride
Anxiety, 206–207,215
Aspirin, for body temperature elevation, 133
Autoimmune response, 20
Automobile, hand controls, 114–115
Autonomic nervous system, 180
Azathioprine, 64,244
  efficacy, 64

  side effects, 64
  teratogenicity, 64

B cell, function, 20
Babinski sign, 25
Baclofen
  dosage, 59
  in spasticity, 59
Baking, 123–124
Bathing, 115–118,140
  getting in and out of tub, 115
  testing temperature of water, 115
  wash mit in, 118
Bed sores, see Decubitus ulcers
Bedroom, 126–128
  bed, 127
Bentyl, see Dicyclomine
Betadine, 137
Bethanecol chloride, 158
Biofeedback, 90
  bowel incontinence and, 175
  as refinement of exercise therapy, 91
  urinary incontinence and, 170
Birth control, 194–195
Bladder, urinary, see Urinary bladder
Bladder dysfunction, 150–170
  diagnosis of, 151–157
  cytoscopy in, 157
  intravenous pyelogram/urogram in, 155–156

263

Bladder dysfunction (*contd.*)
   residual urine determination in, 153–155
      ultrasound in, 155
      urinalysis in, 152–153
      urine culture in, 153
      urodynamic studies in, 156
   emptying disorder, 151,158–162
   management of, 157–163
      emptying disorder, 158–162
      "mixed" type disorder, 162–163
      storage disorder, 157
   "mixed" type disorder, 151,162–163
   storage disorder, 150,157
   surgical procedures in, 166–167
      cystostomy, 166–167
      sphincterotomy, 167
      transurethral resection, 167
Bladder training, 158
Body temperature, 80,132
   elevation, non-exercise related, 132–133
   exercise and, 81
Bonine, *see* Meclazine hydrochloride
Bowel dysfunction, 170–176
   biofeedback in management of, 175
Braces
   evaluation, 107
   leg, 85
   purpose, 107
Brainstem auditory evoked potential, 33,37

Calcium, 70
Cane, types of, 110
Car, *see* Automobile
Carbamazepine, 60,134,183–184
   dosage, 61
   indications for, 61
   side effects, 61
Carbohydrates, 69–70
Carpel tunnel syndrome, 47
Catheter
   condom, 168,169
   external, 168
   urinary, 142
Catheterization
   diagnostic, 154
   indwelling, 163–166, *see also* Indwelling catheter
   intermittent, 159–162, *see also* Intermittent catheterization
   self, 161,162
Central nervous system, anatomy, 13
Cerebellum, plaques in, 46
Cerebrospinal fluid examination, 37–38
Charcot's disease, 197
Chlordiazepoxide, with clinidium, 63
Clinidium, with chlordiazepoxide, 63
Clinitron bed, 139
Clonus, 46
Cobra venom, 244
Colchicine, 66
Color blindness, 33
Colostrum, hyperimmune, bovine, 244
Computer-assisted tomography, 35

SUBJECT INDEX

Constipation, 47,131,171–172
  diet and, 77
  drug-induced, 172
  laxatives in, 172
Contraceptive pill, 194
Contracture
  defined, 140
  surgical correction of, 141
Cooking, 123–124
Coordination
  loss of, 87–89
    manifestations of, 87–88
    spontaneous remission of, 87
    therapeutic exercise in, 88–89
Copolymer, 60,244
Council of State Administrators of Vocational Rehabilitation, 232
Counseling, 218
  family, 212
  group, 211–212
  services, 256,257
Crutch, forearm, 110
Cyclophosphamide, 64,244
  efficacy, 64
  side effects, 65
Cyclosporin, 64,244
Cylert, see Pemoline
Cystospaz, see Hyoscyamine
Cystostomy, 166–167
Cytoxan, see Cyclophosphamine

Dacomed Snap-Gauge band, 181
Dantrium, see Dantrolene sodium
Dantrolene sodium
  side effects, 59
  in spasticity, 59
Depression, 38,202

Decubitus ulcers
  cause of, 82,135
  prevention of, 135–137
  treatment, 137–139
Dexamethasone, dosage, 58
Diabetes mellitus, 131
Diazepam
  side effects, 59
  in spasticity, 59
Dicyclomine bromide, 62
Dicyclomine hydrochloride, dosage, 63
Diet, 67–78
  constipation and, 77
  essential food elements, 68–72
  reducing, 72–75
  urinary tract infection and, 76–77
Dilantin, see Phenytoin
Disability, WHO definition, 230
Dishes, washing, 123
Ditropan, see Oxybutynin
Dizziness, 48
Dogs, 22–23
Double vision, 27

Elavil, see Amitriptyline
Electroencephaly, 33
Emotional lability, 201
Employment, 229–237
Esophagostomy, 143
Euphoria, 38,201
Exacerbations, pseudo, 46,133
Exercise, 131–132
  after acute attack of weakness, 82
  backlying, 96–100,104–107
  balance, 95

Exercise (*contd.*)
  biofeedback, 90
    as refinement of, 91
  body temperature and, 81
  facelying, 92–94
  facilitation, 90
  following removal of splint or cast, 87
  hands and knees position, 94–96
  heavy resistance, 83
  passive, 139–141
  personal regimen, 91–103
    number of activities in, 91
  PROM, 139
  push-ups, 94
  sit-ups, 97
  stretching, 104–107
  as treatment for multiple sclerosis, 79
  under water, 85, 92
  weights in, 92, 93, 99
  in wheelchair, 89, 100–102

Familial essential tremor, 28
Family relationships, 204–206
  with children, 221–222
  with parents, 219–221
  with spouse, 223–227
Fatigue, 144–145
  sexual dysfunction and, 184–185
Fats, 70
Fecal incontinence collector, 175
Fertility, 194
Fibrous contractures, 48
Flavoxate hydrochloride, 62
Flicker fusion test, 35
Foley catheter, 163
Food elements, essential, 68–72

Forearm crutch, 110
Furadantin, *see* Nitrofurantoin

Gantanol, *see* Sulfonamides
Gantrisin, *see* Sulfonamides
Gastrostomy, 143
Glaucoma, anticholinergic agents and, 157
Grab bars, 115

Half-Fare Program for the Handicapped, 237
Handicap, WHO definition, 230
Hiprex, *see* Methenmine hippurate
Hollister collector, 175
Home health services, 254–255
Homemaker services, 258
Homosexuality, 194
Hoyer lift, 140
Hyoscyamine, 62
Hyperbaric oxygen, 244
Hypertension, 131

Imipramine, 62
  dosage, 63
Immune response, 20
Immune system, 20–21
Immunoglobulin, 21, 244
Immunosuppressive agents, 64–65
Impairment, WHO definition, 230
Imuran, *see* Azathioprine, 64
Incontinence, 47
Indiral, *see* Propranolol
Indwelling catheters, 164–166
  care of, 164–166

SUBJECT INDEX

indications for use of, 163–164
stone formation and, 166
urinary tract infection and, 165
Interferon, 66,244
Intermittent catheterization, 159–162
  goals, 159–160
  technique, 160–162
Intravenous pyelogram/urogram, 155–156
Iodine, 70
Iron, 70
Isoniazid, and tremor, 60

Kimura blink reflex, 37
Kitchen, 119–123
  canisters, 120
  cooking utensils, organization of, 120
  counter top height, 120
  design of, 119–120
  gadgets, useful, 125–126
  refrigerator, 122
  sink, 122–123
  storage space, 121–122
  work surfaces, 120

Laxatives, 172
Lhermitte sign, 28,44
Lifeguard rail, 115
Linoleic acid, 71–72
Lioresal, see Baclofen
Lymphocytapheresis, 244
Lymphoid irradiation, 244

Macrodantin, see Nitrofurantoin
Magnesium, 70
Magnetic resonance imaging, 34
Masturbation, 184
Meclazine hydrochloride, 61
Medicaid, 251,254
Medicare, 251,253
Medical Rehabilitation Research and Training Center of Multiple Sclerosis, 234
Memory, 200
Mentor Hold-Free Glans Cap, 168
Methenamine hippurate, 64
  vitamin C and, 64
Minerals, 70–71
Misstique, 168
Monoclonal antibodies, 66,244
Multiple sclerosis
  ACTH in, 54,57
  age of onset, 29
  anxiety and, 206–207,215
  ataxia and, 46
  autoimmunity and, 199,240
  bladder dysfunction in, 45,47, 150–170, see also Bladder dysfunction
  body temperature in, 80
  bowel function in, 45,47,170–176
  braces in, 85
  canine distemper and, 53
  clonus and, 46
  cognitive deficits and, 38
  color blindness in, 33
  common symptoms, 26
  constipation and, 47
  course of the disease, 49–51
  CSF immunoglobulin in, 21
  depression and, 202
  diabetes mellitus in, 131

268 SUBJECT INDEX

Multiple sclerosis (contd.)
  diagnosis, 17,25–42
    brainstem auditory evoked response in, 37
    cerebrospinal fluid examination in, 37–38
    computer-assisted tomography in, 35
    differential, 26–29
    electroencephalography in, 25
    electromyography in, 35
    emotional turbulence following, 216
    of exacerbation, 40–41
    grieving following, 217
    informing patient of, 41–42
    magnetic resonance imaging in, 35
    nerve conduction velocity testing in, 35
    neurophysiological tests in, 33–35
    patient's response to, 204, 209,216,217
    psychological tests in, 38–39
  dizziness and, 48
  dogs and, 22–23
  dorsal column stimulation and, 244
  double vision in, 27
  effect on hearing, 48
  emotional impact of, 190
  emotional lability in, 201
  employment opportunities, 229–237
  endurance training in, 83
  etiology, 13–23,239
    virus infection and, 8
  euphoria and, 201
  exacerbation, 40–41
    pseudo, 46
  exercise as treatment for, 79,131–132
  family counseling, 212
  family relationships in, 219–227
  fatigue and, 39,48,144–145
  fibrous contractures, 48
  frequency of primary symptoms, 44
  gait disturbance in, 27
  genetic factors, 9–10
  group counseling in, 211–212
  heat intolerance in, 133
  hypertension in, 131
  impact on patient's family, 204–206, see also Family relationships
  incidence, 2,4
  individual counseling in, 210
  intellectual changes in, 200
  life expectancy and, 147
  linoleic acid and, 71–72
  lymphocytes in plaques, 20
  memory and, 200
  mood disturbances and, 38
  motor symptoms, 134
  "nerve blocks" in, 86
  nonambulant individual in, 89
  nursing care in, 129–145
  optic nerve inflammation in, 27
  orientation groups, 209–210
  parental guilt in, 221
  performing everyday activities with, 109–128
    bathing, 115–118
    cooking and baking, 123–124

dressing, 127–128
driving a car, 114
oral hygiene, 119
shampooing, 119
shaving, 119
toileting, 118
using the bathroom sink, 118–119
using the kitchen, 119–126
walking, 109–111
personality and, 201
the development of, 198
pregnancy and, 51,217
pressure sores, 48, see also Decubitus ulcer
prevalence, 4,43
psychological aspects, 197
psychological support in, 209
psychotherapy in, 189
rest in, need for, 132
secondary symptoms, 48–49
self-esteem and, 203
sensory symptoms, 134
sexual dysfunction in, 179–187, see also Sexual dysfunction
sexuality, 171–195, see also Sexuality
signs and symptoms, 43–51
skin as a protective agent in, 134–137
social adaptations in, 188,215–227
spasticity in, 84–87
swallowing and, 49,142–143
symptoms, 133–134
temperature and the development of, 43
therapy, 239–245
  experimental, 239–245
toxins and, 19
trauma and, 51
treatment
  with diet, 67–78
  drug therapy, 53–66
  immunosuppressive therapy, 64–65
  physical therapy, 79–107
urinary symptoms in, 147, see also Bladder dysfunction
  treatment of, 62
urinary tract infection, 49
verbal fluency and, 200
viruses and, 19,21–22
visual symptoms, 134
vitamin deficiency and, 19
walking in, 82
weakness in, 81–83
Myelin, 14
Myelography, 37

Nalidixic acid, 63
Nardil, see Phenelezine
National Institute of Handicapped Research, 232
National Multiple Sclerosis Society, 219,232
  employment activities, 234
Negram, see Nalidixic acid
Nerve blocks, 86–87
Nerve impulse conduction, 14,15
Neurogenic bladder, 148
Nitrofurantoin, 63
Node of Ranvier, 15
Nursing care, 129–145
  nurse as interpreter of technical information, 129

Nutrition, 67–78,130–131, *see also* Diet
  supplemental, 76
Nystagmus, 25

Optic nerve inflammation, 27, 47
Oral hygiene, 119
Oxybutynin, dosage, 63
Oxybutynin chloride, 62

Passive range of motion, 139
Pemoline, 62
Penile prosthesis, 182–183
Personality, multiple sclerosis and, 201
Phenelezine
  dosage, 61
  indications for, 61
  side effects, 61
Phenytoin, 60,134,184
  dosage, 61
  side effects, 61
Phosphorus, 70
Physiatrists, 144
Physical therapy, 79–107, *see also* Exercise
  evaluation of, 92
Plasma cell, 16
Plasmapheresis, 244
Portascoot cart, 185
Povidone iodine, 137
Prednisone, 57,244
  dosage, 58
Pregnancy, 51,217
Pressure sores, 48

Pro-Banthine, *see* Propantheline bromide
Projects with Industry, 234
Propantheline bromide, 62
  dosage, 63
Propranolol, tremor and, 60
Prosthesis, penile, 182
Protein, 69
Pseudoexacerbation, 46,133
Psychotherapy, 198
Pulleys, 99

Radioisotope renal/residual urine study, 154–155
Rehabilitation, defined, 143
Rehabilitation Act (1973), 232
Rehabilitation services, 231
Rehabilitation Services Administration, 232
  Projects with Industry, 234
Residual urine determination, 153–155

Sandimmune, *see* Cyclosporin
Scooter, 113
Self-esteem, 203,207–208
Sexual dysfunction, 179–187
  fatigue and, 184–185
  neurophysiological changes and, 180–184
  psychological aspects of, 187–191
Sexuality, 177–195
Shampooing, 119
Shaving, 119
Sign, vs symptom, 25
Skin, 134–137

SUBJECT INDEX

Social adaptations, 215–227
Social Security Administration, 251
Social Security Disability Insurance, 233,251,253
Solu-Medrol, dosage, 58
Somatosensory evoked potential, 33
Spasticity, 84–87,140
  baclofen in, 59
  cause of, 84
  deformities and, 85–86
  drug therapy for, 84–85
  leg braces and, 85
  "nerve blocks" in, 86
  pharmacotherapy in, 59
Sphincterotomy, 167
Splints, purpose, 107
State agencies, rehabilitation services, 231
Stress, in the etiology of multiple sclerosis, 200
Sulfonamides, 63
Supplemental Security Income, 251,253
Swallowing, 49,142–143
Swimming pool, exercise in, 85,92
Symmetrel, *see* Amantidine
Symptom, vs sign, 25

T cell
  effector, 20
  function, 20
  regulatory, 20
Talking books, 258
Tegretol, *see* Carbamazepine
Temperature, body, 80, *see also* Body temperature
Thymosin, 244
Tizanidine, in spasticity, 59

Tofranil, *see* Imipramine
Toileting, 118
  bidet unit, 118
  raised toilet seat, 118
Total lymphoid irradiation, 244
Toxins, 19
Trans-aid, 140
Transfer factor, 244
Transfer tub bench, 116
Transurethral resection, 167
Tremor, propranol in, 60
Tricyclic antidepressants, side effects, 62
Trimethroprim, 63
Trimpex, *see* Trimethoprim
Tylenol, *see* Acetaminophen

Ultrasound, 155
Urecholine, 63
Urinalysis, 152–153
Urinary bladder, normal function, 148
Urinary catheter, *see* Catheter
Urinary disorders, 148–150
  frequency, 149
  hesitancy, 149
  incontinence, *see* Urinary incontinence
  nocturia, 150
  urgency, 149
  urinary tract infection, *see* Urinary tract infection
Urinary incontinence, 149–150, *see also* Bladder dysfunction
  biofeedback and, 170
  products for managing, 167–170
  diaper-type, 170

Urinary incontinence (*contd.*)
    drainage bags, 168–170
    female collection devices, 168
    male external catheters, 168
Urinary symptoms, treatment of, 62
Urinary tract
    anatomy, 149
    infection, *see* Urinary tract infection
Urinary tract infection, 49, 150
    cranberry juice in, 131
    diet and, 76–77
    prophylaxis, 63–64
Urine, culture of, 153
Urispas, *see* Flavoxate hydrochloride
Urodynamic studies, 156

Valium, *see* Diazepam
Viruses, 19, 21–22
    canine distemper, 22
    measles, 22
    slow, 23
Visual evoked potential, 33
Vitamin A, 71
Vitamin B-complex, 71
Vitamin C, 71
    with methenamine, 64
Vitamin D, 71
Vitamins, 71
Vitamin deficiency, 19

Walker, 110
Walking, aids, 109–111
Weakness, 81–83
    arms, 81–82
    cause of, 81
    continuous, 81
    cuff, 93, 99, 100
    cyclical, 81
    legs, 81
    speed of process, 81
Weights
    in exercise, 92, 93, 99
    plate, 100
    pulleys with, 99
Wheelchair
    exercise in, 89, 100–102
    motorized, 113
    part-time use, 111
    seat cushion, 113
    selection of, 111–113
    sports, 114
    types of, 112